Culture and Psychopathology

Georgi Onchev

Culture and Psychopathology

The Anthropology of Mental Illness

Bibliographic Information published by the Deutsche Nationalbibliothek
The Deutsche Nationalbibliothek lists this publication in the Deutsche Nationalbibliografie; detailed bibliographic data is available online at http://dnb.d-nb.de.

Library of Congress Cataloging-in-Publication Data
A CIP catalog record for this book has been applied for at the Library of Congress.

On the cover: Handprints in Cueva de las Manos (Cave of the hands), Argentina, dating back to around 7,500 BCE (Courtesy to Getty Images).

The first edition of this book is in Bulgarian, Riva Publishers, Sofia, 2017. Translated by Sophia Kleinsasser, Mariana Schipkowenska, and Georgi Onchev.

ISBN 978-3-631-79461-6 (Print)
E-ISBN 978-3-631-79467-8 (E-PDF)
E-ISBN 978-3-631-79468-5 (EPUB)
E-ISBN 978-3-631-79469-2 (MOBI)
DOI 10.3726/b15853

© Peter Lang GmbH
Internationaler Verlag der Wissenschaften
Berlin 2019
All rights reserved.

Peter Lang – Berlin · Bern · Bruxelles · New York · Oxford · Warszawa · Wien

All parts of this publication are protected by copyright. Any utilisation outside the strict limits of the copyright law, without the permission of the publisher, is forbidden and liable to prosecution. This applies in particular to reproductions, translations, microfilming, and storage and processing in electronic retrieval systems.

This publication has been peer reviewed.

www.peterlang.com

To the ancestors

Foreword to the Bulgarian Edition

The book *Culture and Psychopathology: The Anthropology of Mental Illness* by Prof. Georgi Onchev sets itself the ambitious task of exploring the relationship between human culture and the phenomenon of mental illness, that which has embarrassed, fascinated, and challenged educated minds throughout the centuries. Various manifestations of this phenomenon are examined in specific cultural contexts, presented with notable competence, and illustrated with memorable descriptions of clinical cases. In search of insight, the author resorts to different theoretical schools and with ease crosses the borders of several scientific disciplines, including psychiatry, psychology, anthropology, neurophysiology, history, and paleontology.

With such inter-disciplinary scope, it is no surprise that the book is full of highly varied information, which is neatly organized and systematized in a reader-friendly way. The text is displayed within the tense conceptual field between the universal truths of human nature and its unexpected idiosyncratic manifestations that elude generic categorization, refute orderly explanatory constructions, and require hermeneutic immersion. The accepted phenomenological approach, likely provoked by the author's clinical practice in different cultural communities, attaches a specific density to the text, a non-final intonation, and theoretical openness which resonates within the context of the late-modern mind's restless meta-scientific quests.

The book and its author have many merits—the capacity to present a highly specialized subject in an intelligible, absorbing, and simultaneously profound manner; respectable erudition and academic self-discipline; and the notable skill of handling different domains of knowledge, among others. The most remarkable quality, however, is the author's concern both for the reader—who is carefully led into quite unknown and still frightening territory—as well as for his protagonists, the mentally ill.

All told, I believe that this book will be of interest not just to students of psychiatry, psychology, and anthropology, but also to a broader circle of readers who are excited by the wretched and admirable destiny of being human.

Prof. Haralan Alexandrov, Dr.Sc. anthropology

Contents

1 Introduction: Heritage and Phenomena 11

2 Culture: Essence and Dimensions 19
   2.1 Elusiveness in Culture 20
   2.2 Cultural Axes 26

3 Cultural Context at Home: the Bulgarian Odysseus 33
   3.1 Antinomies of the Bulgarian Mentality 33
   3.2 Traumatic Memory and an "Optimistic Theory" 39

4 Psychopathology: Essence and Manifestation 45
   4.1 The Syndrome 47
      Anxiety 49
      Depression 49
      Mania 50
      Acute psychosis 51
      Chronic psychosis 52
      Delirium 53
      Dementia 53
   4.2 Diagnosis and Case Formulation 55

5 The Culture-Psychopathology Relationship 61
   5.1 Historical Steps of Interweaving 62
   5.2 Symptom Formation 70

6 Mysticism and Psychopathology 75
   6.1 Religion and Psychopathology 76
   6.2 The Paranormal and Psychopathology 84

7 Spirit Possession States 91
7.1 Clinical Cases from Pemba Island 92
7.2 Bulgarian Analogues of Possession 97

8 Schizophrenia and Culture 105
8.1 Epidemiology 107
8.2 Clinical Picture 110
8.3 Course and Outcome 116

9 Affective Disorder, Anxiety, and Culture 123
9.1 Depression and Anxiety 124
9.2 Somatization and Dissociation 131

10 Abnormal Behaviors and Culture 135
10.1 Alcohol and Drugs 135
10.2 Personality and Behavioral Pathologies 140

11 Culture Specific Syndromes 145

12 Treatment and Culture 153

13 Epilogue: After Tomorrow 163

List of Figures 167

List of Tables 169

References 171

1 Introduction: Heritage and Phenomena

> Where do we come from? What are we? Where are we going?
>
> *P. Gauguin*

Over 6 million years ago pre-humans and pre-chimpanzees separated and took different roads of evolution, which remained relatively slow until some 11,000 years ago. Modern homo sapiens appeared around 60,000 years ago, and 20,000 years later the Neanderthal man had already started believing in the supernatural, and thus coping with his fears. Still, it would take another 25,000 more years before Cro-Magnons sewed clothing, made tools, painted, and played—thus creating the ritual foundation of culture.[90] 11,000 years before the present, a transition began from hunting and gathering to farming and settlement, and this occurred at the earliest within the valleys of civilization's great rivers: the Nile, Jordan, Tigris, and Euphrates, all along the so-called Fertile Crescent which stretches between Egypt and Mesopotamia (from the Greek, meaning "between the rivers").[47] Later, encounters with non-threatening strangers were tolerated, and history gained momentum. Food production began 9,000 years ago and the first metal tools were made before some 7,000 years, while the first writings and state administrations appeared around 5,400 years ago (3400 BCE), along the Nile and in Mesopotamia, followed shortly by settlements in China, Mexico, the Andes, and Madagascar. All of them were traditional communities: communes, tribes, chiefdoms, and states. The concentration of many people in one place and cattle-breeding resulted in the transmission of microorganisms from animals to humans, and the advent of infectious diseases. In communities larger than tribes, not all people knew each other, so the need for a common sign of recognition arose to prevent unnecessary killing off arose. Thereby, *shared* rituals and ideologies emerged. These communities were ruled by a chief and their assistants, prototypes of the future bureaucrats—this was a universal model as late as the modern 18th century, when changes were brought on by the Industrial Revolution, public health care, and signs of democracy.

War, "the lethal custom of mankind",[50] has accompanied it throughout history. Probably the most striking feature of human development is its endless violence and ferocity. The main causes for fighting were hunger and territorial struggles for hunting land, especially in the "no man's" ones between separate tribal communities. Fortified cities started being built around 5500 BCE, and around 4000 BCE the horse was domesticated, although it would not be until two millennia later that heavier breeds were selected and used for riding into war or pulling supplies. The wheel was invented around 3000 BCE; the two-wheeled cart—approximately 700 years later. The first civilizational separation between settled farmers and nomadic cattle breeders led to the dark epoch of unceasing raids carried out by nomads against city-states between 2000 and 1500 BCE, and necessitated their defense. After 1500 BCE, human civilizations were already totally militarized, and the power of each kingdom, chiefdom, or empire was measured by its fighting strength. For millennia in succession, nomadic raids of settled communities have shaped history, forming the basis of the migration factors[156] for people. In the Fertile Crescent, continuous bloodshed marked the 13-centuries-long domination of Assyria, ending only after the demolition of its capital Nineveh in the 7th century BCE.

The population growth and inhabitation of the steppes, mainly by nomads, caused a struggle for resources which has since become one of the major engines of history—along with successive challenges and responses leading to civilizations' rise, development, decay, or clashing with one another.[206] Theocratic empires such as Rome and Babylon justified their violence and transformed it into a code of behavior. In the Old Testament, the extermination of everyone that does not belong to the chosen people is heroized, with Joshua himself having slaughtered 31 kings and all the inhabitants of 400 towns while conquering the Canaan land. Between the 4th and 14th centuries of the new era, such conflicts became permanent and bloody. Genghis Khan massacred around 40 million Chinese people in order to clear territories as pasture for his herds.[50] After the 14th century great wars occurred on average every 50 years, with subsequent and lasting treaties which established the state of affairs in peacetime. Just two generations later, this state would change, e.g., a country developing more quickly in economic and demographic terms, now no longer in concord with the situation allotted to it by the previous treaty, signed when it was weak and poor. Besides the two world wars of the 20th century, there were at least five more big wars with a worldwide scope, including the Thirty Years' War, the Seven Years' War, and the Napoleonic Wars. The creation of modern nation states in the 18th and 19th centuries would stimulate further militarism.

There have existed constantly militant cultures, possessed by "constructive paranoia",[47] like some tribes in New Guinea, the Aztecs, the Mayans, and the Incas. In patrilocal societies, with extended families rearing children as a unit, wars were waged not through large-scale battles or by following any rules, but with tactics very much like those of guerilla warfare. The abandonment or killing of frail elderly people in order to spare the burden of care, is still common in many cultures. In the Kaulong tribe of New Britain, there is a custom to ritually strangulate widows,[47] which is accepted by the victims without resistance. Human sacrifice rituals have been known in almost all cultures throughout history, including the First Bulgarian kingdom before the state conversion to Christianity. The forefather of monotheism, Abraham, did not hesitate at all in cutting his son Isaac's throat under the order of God, who held him back at the last moment (Genesis). And infanticide is also common in all cultures, not only because of congenital ailments, but also as a means of controlling population growth. A rough estimate suggests that probably around 15 % of all children in human history have been killed;[50] in England this practice was preserved even into the 19th century. Infanticide is also common in animals, for instance, when a lion kills another lion and its cubs, but not the lionesses, in order for that lion to have cubs with her and not have to care for the others.

Violence in human history has often been the only means for survival: sparing another from violence only makes one a victim of violence. In a fight for resources, violence is moreover the fastest way of getting rich. But it is also genetically predetermined. The human race is an evolutionary branch with an inherited inclination towards domination and hierarchy, especially in males. The closest primates to us genetically are hunters who eat meat and display intraspecies aggression. Only predators kill individuals from their own species, and the most ferocious among them are those at the top of the evolutionary chain—chimpanzees and people. Most people, under certain circumstances, are capable of murder (though most would deny it) and, apart from that, most would even experience pleasure from this act in the right conditions.[50, 90] Human babies are helpless for a relatively long time compared to other mammals' babies; they therefore only have a chance at survival with two parents available. Thus, families generate. The rearing of children requires relative tranquility which, with humans' aggressive nature, may only be guaranteed by a powerful state that can ensure peace, thereby protecting families and offspring. For this reason, all civilizations until only several centuries before now have been exclusively authoritarian. Between 600 BCE and 600 CE, the major religions, i.e., Judaism and its branches, Christianity, Islam, and Buddhism, were born. For the first time, the anti-authoritarian idea that people are equal (at least before God) sneaks in.

Culture appeared with the arousal of self-consciousness and as a response to the need to bear the truth of one's own mortality. It is a dynamic system of rules which ensure *survival* and are transmitted down generations. The development of symbols, rituals, and beliefs had to come to terms with the necessity to cope with the horror of dying. This role was most immediately filled by religion, which is a direct cultural product.⁹⁰, ²⁰⁶ Cultures are over-biological systems, however, they have been formed throughout the course of human evolution by biological and geographical factors, as well as their mutual exchange. There is evidence from archaeological artefacts with radiocarbon dating and written data which talk of a huge cataclysm around 5100 years ago, or around 3100 BCE, altering the borders between land and oceans and forcing people to flee and migrate elsewhere.⁸⁵ It is probable that this refers to the sinking of Atlantis—a myth coming from Plato, Solon, and ancient Egyptian papyruses. At that time, everywhere on the large Afro-Eurasian island, paleolithic people were living in traditional primitive communities, while in Mesopotamia and Egypt, flourishing civilizations simultaneously sprang out. Their common cultural signs were their pride, the legend that they were the heirs of gods, a strict hierarchy, the building of pyramids, walls, and towns, powerful religious cults, depictions of avian humanoids, hieroglyphs, monumental art,⁸⁵ initiation rites, play,⁹⁰ and the myth of eternal return.⁵²

Around 1200 BCE, a new cataclysm, probably set off by a volcanic eruption on Santorini in the Mediterranean, and the tsunamis that followed, caused the flooding and destruction of coastal towns and cultures, with the survivors fleeing to the mainland interior. The coincidence of this date with the Jews' escape from Egypt, led by Moses and Aaron in 1200 BCE, invites the conclusion that the Biblical story of the Red Sea being parted and the water rushing back soon after, consuming the Pharaoh's army (Exodus), documents a real disaster, albeit with the inevitable interpretation of divine involvement.⁸⁵

Besides the mythologies of the civilizations around the two great valleys, the dates of the huge cataclysms in 3100 BCE and 1200 BCE are also significant in the cultural memory of peoples from the other side of the Atlantic Ocean—the Mayans, the Aztecs, and the Incas. According to the Mayan calendar, the year zero was in 3113 BCE, when ships with pale-faced, bearded men wearing turbans and broad dressing gowns arrived from the East. They laid the foundation of the Olmec culture, which, millennia later, in turn would generate the cultures of the Incas, the Aztecs, the Mayans, and the entire cultural belt from Mexico to Peru. Analyzing ancient navigation routes demonstrates many cultural analogies, such as pottery, bricklaying tools, and trepanation, and provides interpretive arguments for the archaic contact that may have existed between cultures across the seas, possibly established in the first place by the Phoenicians crossing the Strait of Gibraltar and reaching the Caribbean Sea.⁸⁵

The direction of the currents and winds, along with cultural transfers (and raids), have always been from East to West: from Asia to Europe, from Africa

Introduction: Heritage and Phenomena   15

and Europe to America, and from America to Asia. There are two approaches to interpreting cultural similarities in different parts of the world. According to isolationists, cultures evolve independently to common civilizational levels, while according to diffusionists, this is achieved by transferring culture traits from place to place. The places, where civilizations have developed totally independently, however, are indeed very few in mankind's history. If no transfers ever took place, many cultures would still be in the primitive communal system— and some still are at present. Thus, modern civilization is the heir of common ancestors from Egypt and Mesopotamia[206] (and probably from Atlantis before them), who dispersed their cultural seeds across the Mediterranean, Europe, and the Americas. Their descendants share an archaic ontology and similar cultural signs like the story of a patriarchal ancestor, strong connections with gods, and the development of writing through common stages: hieroglyphs, cuneiform writing, and letters.

Cultural evolution has created distinctions and borders. For instance, the division of Rome into the Eastern and Western Empires in the 4th century would for centuries onward predetermine the basic civilizational boundaries of the Old World: between Catholicism and Protestantism on one side, and Orthodox Christianity and Islam on the other.[91] The line of this division, which stretches from the border between Russia and Finland in the north to the Western Balkans in the south, has been relatively steady for almost two millennia, particularly in the Balkans, where it passes between the territories of the former Ottoman and Habsburg empires and their national successors. Characteristics of mentality are more influential than those of ideology,[207] and for that reason, political blocks uniting countries from different cultures are artificial;[15, 16] this is also why such countries return to their cultural families after the blocks' disintegration. For example, Bulgaria and the Czech Republic belonged for nearly 50 years (too short a period from a culture-time perspective) to the same ideological space, yet, when both places are assessed according to different cultural dimensions, the Czechs are predictably closer to Germany than Bulgaria.[143] Cultural similarities lead to more lasting alliances than ideological ones, forming civilization groups such as the West, Orthodoxy, Confucianism, or Latino.

When reaching its zenith, each civilization creates the experience of its history coming to a final end.[118, 206] In the last millennium, the West played a role in human development analogous to that of Mesopotamia several millennia earlier. The influence of Western civilization increased from the 9th century until the 20th century, and afterwards began to decrease. The collapse of ideologies causes the return to local, traditional, national, or religious sources of identity. Though its victorious position after the Cold War, the West has provoked anti-Western attitudes and the embrace of Asian cultural ideas, including those of Islam, and all the more so with its attempts to "export" liberal values. New boundaries have formed around the oppositions between the West and Islam, the Third World, China, or Eurasia (or between Islam and the rest), as well as within countries where inner dividing lines or orientations tend to oscillate.[91]

A paradoxical *cyclicity* is present in this cultural development. After a secular and scientific period of flourishing, there is a return to religion as a major cultural identifier and to war as the core of history and a proven path to power and wealth. Authoritarian rules are followed by a return to the egalitarianism of ancient hunter-gatherers with their long talks around the fire; communism is an eschatological and prophetic repetition of early Christianity;[94] and what follows the disappointment of democracy is a new authoritarianism.[63] The transition from the collective values of traditional cultures to the individualism of modernity gives way to existential insecurity, loneliness, and the need for renewed collective unity and transcendent order, and even new forms of identities (Chapter 13).

The codes of the past live on in the psyche. The ways we eat, feel, think, entertain ourselves, or cope with fears are steeped in the rules that governed our upbringing. Newborns have no culture; instead, babies encounter it in the first instants of life through diapering, feeding, and touch. Psychopathology, an extremity in itself of normal psychological processes (Chapter 4), is an *epigenetic product* of cultural evolution. Its *phenomena* (not its causes, which are usually unknown) are modeled by culture through the filtering of psychological and biological morbid signals in the process of symptom formation. Traces of the past participate in symptom formation and contribute to its understanding. The depreciation of the past, along with guilty and hypocritical refrains for turning back to it, is itself a culture-specific characteristic of the *hypometropia*[143] dimension, or shortsightedness, as described by the Bulgarian cultural anthropologist M. Minkov. As W. Faulkner writes, "the past is never dead. It's not even past". Psychopathology does not emerge out of nothingness, but rather sets foot on human history and culture like a dwarf on the shoulders of a giant from U. Eco's interpretation[51] of the medieval metaphor. The roots of psychopathology exist within the normal psyche, and the normal psyche is rooted in culture. Psychopathology and culture are similar in that they are both over-biological interpretative systems, and not ontological realities (Chapter 5). The clinical and anthropological nuances of their mutual interweaving can facilitate deeper insight into each of them: understanding one system is facilitated by its reflection in the other, and by the modes of interaction between both of them. The ambition to achieve such understanding cannot rely on trivial academic exercises, but must be a free creative journey that crosses the borders of different disciplines, genres, dogmas and expressions. My view on the topic has been formed by a long and unfinished journey.

2 Culture: Essence and Dimensions

> Although changed, I arise the same (Eadem mutato resurgo)
>
> *Words of the Spiral, by J. Bernoulli*

Culture is social heredity. Apart from a plethora of academic definitions, the preservation of human experience is culture's basic feature. It is a system of *shared meanings* for the interpretation of this experience with the ultimate goal of survival and confidence. Societal DNA spares the necessity of each new generation re-inventing the rules for living; instead, they can absorb them from their ancestors, thus saving energy for development. As the great 4th-century Arab physician Rhazes writes, the experience of one person compared to everyone from all the ages, resembles "a trickle of water, flowing into a big river".[14] Culture protects against the loss of objects and anxiety in the face of the unknown, much like the presence of parents calms a baby in the dark. It creates, for a group of people, a collective system of rules that encompasses attitudes, beliefs, values, and norms shared by all members, ensuring their survival and being passed from generation to generation. For this reason, cultural traits remain stable over time. Though the potential for change exists, these traits are part of an essentially conservative system with an evolutionary sense which imposes a slow pace of change, never altering the basic aspects of the system. The modern era, however, has accelerated this speed (Chapter 13) and, thence, culture undergoes changes and *arises the same*.

In his *Histories*, Herodotus[220] describes how King Darius I of Persia (5th century BCE) asked some Hellenes how much they would want to be paid in order to eat the bodies of their dead fathers. They replied that they would not do this for anything in the world. Then, with the same Hellenes observing, Darius asked some Indians, who had been known to eat their dead fathers, how much they would want to be paid in order to burn the bodies of their fathers when they died. The Indians cried out and begged him not to even mention such a thing. "Custom is the king over everything", the father of history comments, citing the ancient Greek lyric poet Pindar. What Darius, Pindar, and Herodotus called custom, is in fact culture, while "king over everything" is one of its shortest definitions.

The determinative features of culture are those that we are usually unaware of.[83, 106] They are so deeply embedded that no formal rules exist for them—they are taken for granted. They do not teach us explicitly, for instance, how far away to stand from the person we are conversing with, or when it is inappropriate to laugh. Nevertheless, we usually do not make mistakes, if our childhood was spent in the same culture, when it comes to talking and laughing. In a given culture, the *unwritten rules* are pivotal. They are the most stable over time and the hardest to break. Any attempt to break them causes anxiety and the mobilization of group protection.

2.1 Elusiveness in Culture

The *origin* of culture is associated with evolutionary biology and psychological processes. The psyche arose out of the necessity to communicate, and the moment when man realized his own mortality may be considered as the birth of culture. Culture makes the idea of death bearable through rituals and symbols, and this explains why it is not an accurate reflection of reality. Psychological cultural components, such as religion, tales, and fantasies, distort reality in a creative manner and for the purposes of adaptation. There are signs that at the time of its genesis, homo sapiens was surrounded by about 15 other humanoids who did not survive, yet we lack evidence of their extermination.[47] The sole survival of homo sapiens was due to the fact that our most distant ancestor created culture—stories about prevailing, transcending, and continuing one's life beyond death. Believing in a kind of spiritual protection made humans bolder both as hunters and in the struggle to survive. The First World War gave rise to the expression that, at machine-gun point, there are no atheists. People's transition to settlements increased their confidence in beliefs and explanations about the world, and life after death, simply because they were shared by more followers. The funeral customs of different cultures over millennia have, in fact, represented a symbolic denial of death: burying alive servants and concubines, and even a whole army of terracotta warriors and horses with the Chinese emperors; or the march of Gilgamesh, in the ancient Sumerian epic, in search of immortality after the death of his beloved friend Enkidu.

Culture includes subjective elements, social rules, and material traces of ethnic, racial, religious, or social groups of people. Living in groups helps them to survive and cope with the problems of biological imperatives like finding food and reproduction, depending on the specifics of different social or climatic environments. In the Middle East, for instance, it is difficult to breed pigs because they are fed with grain, making them competitors for human food, and besides, they do not gain weight as cattle do in the region. For this reason, the religious ban on eating pork in Judaism and Islam has its practical grounds in geographical conditions, and only post hoc was transformed into religious dogma.[143] Living together also imposes the development of norms in human relationships, with a reverse action on biology via natural selection. Despite cultural differences, there are five moral norms that make adaptation and collective living easier, and they are considered to be universal:[181] submission to authority, reciprocity, care, social responsibility, and solidarity.

Besides the biological, culture also has its psychological foundations. Self-knowledge and neuroplasticity create rules, hierarchies, and lessons on how to live that relieve existential insecurity, ensure support by the group, re-confirm the picture of the world through common views, ensure the automaticity of daily life with a dynamic construction of the experience, and, in general, establish order. Culture masters global chaos by creating order. The main *components* of culture are subjective, and they are inter-linked as in a syndrome. They include values, norms, beliefs, attitudes, self-perception, cognitive abilities, behaviors, and stereotypes—all of them shared. Culture, however, is not an individual construct, but a group one, i.e., referring to a tribe, horde, ethnicity, nation, sub-society, or gang. Intuitive assumptions about the world and mythical stories are usually shared by all members of the group, but the group's norms, due to individual differences, are not. The fewer of them who do not share it, the higher the probability for such members to be regarded as exhibiting some deviation or even pathology. The social lesson of culture is: when in doubt, copy your age peers and members of your gender group.

This is a lesson learned during childhood by assimilating the external rules of behavior (*socialization*) and the essential, unconscious aspects of culture that are internalized like "second nature" during subsequent development (*enculturation*). In this process of learning, the roles of parents, clans, communities, organizations such as the pioneers or scouts, churches, schools, neighborhoods, or bands vary according to the context. The slower a culture changes, and the more extended the families are within it, the higher the probability that these lessons will be taught by parents or the elderly; while the faster a culture changes and the more nuclear families are, the higher the probability that children will learn them from their peers. Childhood "democracy" is inherent to times of change and rebellion. Generational conflict resembles a test of paradigm checking, yet not in a scientific context but in a cultural one: that which is transient, lacking any enduring cultural roots, is eliminated, while that which sustains rebellion is re-endorsed. Long hair, rock and roll, free love, drugs, and anti-establishment movements, after just one generation, became known as the culture of "old folks".

As *Pravda* newspaper ponderously lectures: "Rock and roll has the right to exist, but only if it is melodious, instructive, and well performed".[108] Culture applies the same justification to rebellion towards itself—making it melodious, instructive, and performed in the right manner.

Values refer to what is important for people: money, glory, family, religion. *Norms* refer to what, according to the people, should or should not be done, e.g., not drinking alcohol during Ramadan. They reflect values, but only in the sense that we expect them from others, or they reflect what we would like to see in them. This does not necessarily coincide with what we expect from ourselves, thus creating a cultural double standard—the difference between what we value personally and in others. *Beliefs* reflect our agreement with certain claims. Certain beliefs that are deeply rooted in culture, such as belief in God, or in the role the common cold plays in causing diseases in Bulgarian culture, are stable over time. *Attitudes* reflect what people like or dislike. *Self-perception* reflects the average level of satisfaction we have with ourselves, e.g., how happy or unhappy we feel. *Cognitive abilities* reflect the potential of our cognitive apparatus, through which we discover and understand phenomena within ourselves and in the world. Different lifestyles can stimulate the development of some instruments that make up this apparatus, at the expense of others. In many cultures, for instance, intellectual success is not of as great importance as it is in developed countries. That is why, despite significant individual variations, differences in average levels of cognitive abilities also exist between nations. *Behaviors* are a set of actions and mannerisms related to changes in the environment or in the body that can be objectively observed in contrast to inner experiences. Cultural differences in behaviors can be manifested, for instance, by the indexes of murders and traffic accidents.

Stereotypes are generalized collective descriptions of groups of people, either strangers or close ones.[143] They have a plain evolutionary basis: we like those that are close to us, and we are suspicious of others. Stereotypes are usually polarizing and homogenized, and they tend to reproduce themselves and gain endorsement in the face of threats or their violation. We all hold sustainable notions from childhood, such as the sentiment that grown boys do not cry, or that girls do not practice arm wrestling. These generalized notions are commonly applied to outsiders, while individual distinctions are commonly taken into account within the group itself—hence, we appear to be diverse, while others look uniform. Generalizations about ourselves and others cause a peculiar cognitive distortion—you see what you believe in. In this way, in cultures where honor is valued, the norms of violence and bloody revenge are sustained. Culture is an inert system and it holds up many stereotypes and magical beliefs long after the reasons behind them have been left to history—this is the *time difference*[143] between culture and history. The formation of stereotypes passes through selective attention, assessment of the relevance of stimuli to our life, formation of categories, attribution of qualities, and consolidation into semantic memory. A prejudice is a preliminary judgment about someone based on the grounds of his or her group affiliation. The cognitive component of prejudice is a stereotype towards the relevant group, while its affective component includes feelings based on personal experience with people from that group. Discrimination is the refusal of rights or privileges (which we otherwise acknowledge for ourselves) to others due to their group affiliation. It is at the core of the "isms" (such as racism or sexism) at the group or organizational level.

These components are united into a cultural matrix, which in turn supports the behaviors which create it, and eventually support it in a reciprocal manner. It embraces the symbols that we share in order to understand one another, and collectively programs our thinking so that we can reliably and consistently discriminate against individuals belonging to one group, and not another one. The capacity for such discrimination on a conscious level is frequently explained by rational categorization, but, in essence, it is an attitude that is unconscious and absorbed very early on—disguised as a rational view of life, cultural binoculars onto the world. Culture is the way things are done in the *daily round* ("here, that's the way it is"), e.g., what to eat and how to eat, whether to use cutlery or eat with fingers, who starts to eat first, sitting at the table or on the floor, or lying down, viewing belching as an obscene act or accepting it as a praise for the cook. In Africa, for example, it is not reasonable to ask questions to which yes is a possible reply because this is precisely what you will receive as an answer. This is not lying, but a display of politeness and the certainty that it would be insulting not to get a yes. Culture is a learned system, an abstraction that cannot be touched, although its manifestations may be concrete and visible, e.g., the Japanese tea ceremony or flower arranging.

The carriers of culture are different groups of people. Nations are not ethnically, socially, or religiously homogeneous, and, for this reason, any assessments of provisional national cultures are indeed relative. When people from different religions live together for a long time, they share common, or very close, cultures, like Muslim and Orthodox Christian Arabs in Israel, or Orthodox Christians and Muslims in Bulgaria. Totalitarianism, being short-lived, failed to generate huge cultural changes, and, soundly, after its collapse, every country returned to the cultural bosom of older identities, such as Orthodoxy, Catholicism, and Islam.

Another carrier is race, despite the political correctness of its depreciation. It is an important construct, yet it is not black-and-white, but rather polythetic.

Race determines essential genetic differences and genetic clustering which are the basis for such anatomical differences as brain, genitalia, or muscle size, bone structure, and the ratio between the lengths of the index and the ring fingers (2D:4D), as well as enzyme and physiological differences, with consequential peculiarities of behavior and predispositions to different diseases. Japanese women, for instance, have low bone density and are more prone to osteoporosis, but nevertheless, have fewer fractures.[133] Physiological differences also exist in perceptions, i.e., optical illusions are not perceived in the same way in different cultures. Similar to the influence of early individual experiences on brain neuroplasticity, cultural styles also affect some biological characteristics. Individual biological differences, however, are much more diverse than group ones. Groups may not live together, but nevertheless can be carriers of cultural similarities, as with the disabled or football fans, or in the fashion world, corporate culture, or gay culture. The trend towards cultural convergence even offers grounds for speculation about a universal culture.

Cultural anthropology originated in the colonial period as a Eurocentric interest towards pre-industrial communities, or as a science dedicated to studying the "life of the natives". Cross-cultural studies check whether what we know about human behavior is also true for other races, cultures, or ways of life. The cross-cultural approach examines whether global truths and principles are universal or culture specific. These studies can be:[133] comparative—assessing differences based usually on one variable; in-depth—explaining the reason behind these differences through other contextual variables; or on an ecological level—with countries and cultures (but not individuals) serving as units for analysis, e.g., G. Hofstede's studies.[87] Cross-validation studies examine whether a measurement from one culture is equivalent and applicable in another one, and this is a problematic area which affects the sense of the examination itself. In assessments by scales, for instance, representatives of collectivistic communities tend to give moderate replies, somewhere in the middle of the response range, in accordance with a cultural tendency not to "stand out", while representatives of individualistic cultures more readily give extreme replies.[181] Even the theoretical foundation of these comparisons has cultural roots in the logical determinism and rationality of Western scientific ideology.[21] The ethnographic approach refers to fieldwork or even living amongst the objects of examination, which is closer to so-called qualitative research,[33, 83] and therefore attempts to overcome the Euro-colonial limitations of cultural anthropology.

While cross-cultural psychology assesses the influence of culture on individual mentality, i.e., using the anthropological framework to assess psychological problems, the examination of the "psychological foundations of culture"[181] is a reverse approach which applies psychological instruments to the assessment and interpretation of culture itself. Cultural meanings are shared cognitions and, in fact, mental phenomena. *Language* and thinking are both influenced by culture and linked to its peculiarities. According to Humboldt, the variety of languages is not a variety of signs or sounds, but of viewpoints about the world.[133] We are all born with similar potential to emit sounds; however, languages teach us to pronounce them differently. Different grammars are, according to the Sapir-Whorf hypothesis, different reflections of reality and ways of sorting acquired knowledge—or it could be said that different languages are different models of *thinking*.[219] Linguistic determinism attributes hidden semantic categories (cryptotypes) to styles of speech, e.g., in psychological gender: the moon, in French, is feminine, while the sun is masculine, while in German, it is the opposite. Anthropologists have also discovered a connection between the tonality of language and type of religion—monotheistic as in Europe and the Middle East, or polytheistic as in the Far East—as well as one between the size of linguistic diversity and geography: larger at the Equator, and decreasing towards the poles.[47]

Nonverbal behavior builds up unconsciously, with culture teaching us the gestures, mimics, intonations, and poses to use. Raised eyebrows are a universal gesture of greeting, but physical touching, on the other hand, provides evidence for broad differences. The Japanese *hai* (yes) along with nodding is a linguistic controller confirming that one is listening—though this may not at all be the case, it is repeated mechanically when communicating.[173] The expression of universal emotions is universal (Chapter 9), however, the rules for their control are specific. This specificity is reflected onto the way signals from others get decoded, as well as social cognition, the latter also being affected by cultural filters, ethnocentrism, emotions, and value judgments. Americans and the Japanese decipher emotional intensity in others' facial expressions in different ways, and control over one's own emotional expression acts decisively in this deciphering,[138] i.e., emotional competence appears to be a complex expectation, where one's own emotional regulation turns into a lens with which to view others.

Cultural differences associated with different methods of swaddling babies, suppressing emotions, and attachment styles are displayed even through temperament, which is, otherwise, biologically determined. Asian babies are, as a rule, quieter and more submissive. Much like the experienced clinician notices not just separate symptoms, but the patient's overall, Gestalt appearance (Chapter 4), the cultural interpretation of psychomotorics reads the underlying inner state according to the nonverbal archetype forming this interpretation. Facial expressions are easier to control than body language, gestures, and alterations of speech. The unclosed, symmetrical, and slightly bent-forward position is a sign of confidence in all cultures, while smiling, calm, and easy gestures made without fidgeting or restlessness, along with flexible movements and fluent speech without lapses, are signs of harmony with the environment and personal maturity in every cultural context.[173]

Distinctions in cognitive styles are present in information processing, categorization, memory, problem solving and decision making, and creativity. Some cultures do not consider abstraction a higher form of cognition. In closed communities with rigid boundaries and experiences of being threatened, the need for a firm social reality causes cognitive closure and the rejection of any information that contradicts this reality. Americans explain the actions of others through their inner states (i.e., a tendency to psychologize), while Indians do so through people's social roles and obligations. When making decisions in individualistic cultures, one usually asks for additional information, while in collectivistic ones, advice from the elderly or a relevant precedent from a more experienced person is sought.[43] Unlike harmonious motor behavior, cognitive creativity is not accepted unequivocally in all cultures. The creative personalities are curious, prefer risks, bear hard work, accept tasks, do not hold dogmas or firm convictions, continually correct their own views, have divergent thinking, and can easily tolerate ambiguity and insecurity. Many cultures do not encourage such qualities, instead requiring their adaptation if not sanctioning them altogether.

2.2 Cultural Axes

Culture may be transformed into a measurable construct by assessing it according to separate traits. The leading trait is the ratio between individual and collective values. In it, cultures are provisionally divided into two large groups: modern and traditional (Tab. 1). Modern culture is indeed sometimes extended through to the postmodern, with its notions of constant change, the fluidity of boundaries, irony, discourse, gender, ecology, relativeness of representations of reality, and fragmentation of authorities and constructs, which, in their extremity, blur the distinction between truths and near-truths—a cognitive distortion referred to by H. Frankfurt as cultural "bullshit".[60] Since postmodernity is still in its *status nascendi*, regarded as a continuation of the existential dimension of modernity, and its consequences on identities and psychopathology are not yet fully understood (Chapter 13), there are no grounds for including it in this division or abandoning the major cultural dichotomy.

In modern cultures, individual values have priority over collective ones, while it is the opposite in traditional cultures. Modern cultures, present mainly

Tab. 1: Basic distinctions between cultures

Traditional cultures	Modern cultures
Collective values	Individual values
Extended families	Nuclear families
Consistent roles	Contradictory roles
Theories of equality	Theories of personal freedom
Group acceptance	Social isolation
Shame	Guilt

in industrialized Western countries, offer powerful stimuli for personal development, liberties, and responsibilities, including personal responsibility over irrational or dangerous behaviors, nuclearization of the family, frequent neglect of care for weak and sick members, social isolation, contradictory expectations of different social roles, and rational interpretations of subjective experiences. In traditional cultures, these characteristics and their consequences have the opposite trend: personal development, liberty, and personal responsibility are not encouraged, families are extended to the size of kin, clan, or tribe, there is unconditional group acceptance, social roles and expectations are consistent and clear, and magical interpretations are common, without focusing on subjective experience. The *locus of control* of one's behavior is external in collectivistic communities, while it is internal in individualistic ones. This division has crucial influence on the other traits of cultures, as well as on illness behavior and the manifestation of psychopathology (Chapter 5).

In his classical research on the "software of the mind", or the group mentality in different people, Hofstede[87] isolates through factor analysis several *dimensions* of culture that explain the majority of variations in behaviors, beliefs, and ways of life. They are: masculinity/femininity, uncertainty avoidance, power distance, individualism/collectivism, and short-term/long-term orientation.

In *masculine* cultures, people tend to sacrifice leisure time for the sake of a professional career, boys and girls are brought up differently (e.g., boys should not cry and look weak or spoiled), there is a sharp contrast in manners between men and women, and over-ambition, strong will, persistence, competition, and workaholism are encouraged. In *feminine* cultures, there is no apparent distinction between the values and mentality of men and women; for instance, men can have jobs associated with care and concern (nurse, babysitter, or preschool teacher), which in turn are not regarded as purely female professions. Feelings, friendships, and pastimes are valued more than success, fame, or wealth.

The *uncertainty avoidance* is a cultural dimension associated with high levels of stress accompanied by impatience, tension, nervousness, and anxiety. As with all cultural phenomena, it is acquired in early childhood, and for this reason, it may be corrected in later life only to some extent. In countries with high levels of uncertainty avoidance, children are not allowed to do many things, e.g., get dirty while playing. The trend to control all aspects of functioning is reproduced and endorsed at later stages—in school, military service or the workplace. Learning through experience is not stimulated, a strict distinction between right and wrong is encouraged, and changes, novelties, and differences are regarded with suspicion.

The *power distance* is an index characterizing the degree to which weaker members of society expect and accept inequality. Inequalities exist everywhere; however, their acceptance varies: in some cultures, external status symbols are not emphasized, while in others they are overtly conspicuous, e.g., designer watches or shoes, or a reserved parking place provided by a corporation. In communities with a high index of power distance, there are significant differences between superiors and subordinates—informal communication on a first-name basis is considered inappropriate, which is in contrast to communities with a low degree of power distance. Subordinates feel, to a considerable degree, dependent on their superiors and do not readily respond to attempts for consultation ("this does not concern me") or assume responsibility.

The *individualism/collectivism* cultural dimension reflects the dominance of values. In collectivistic communities, collective values dominate, i.e., the rights, interests, opinions, and welfare of the family, tribe, team, or fatherland have priority over individual rights, interests, opinions, and welfare. Individual autonomization comes into contradiction with this trend, and is more incidental within cultures where individual values dominate over collective ones. This dimension, frequently referred to as the IC index, is linked to some illnesses and issues with patient autonomy and informed consent (Chapter 13).

The *short-term/long-term orientation* dimension represents the prevailing orientation in the temporal perspective, called also the Confucian dimension. The long-term orientation is dominant in Eastern cultures, denoting effort and the sacrifice of current welfare in the name of some remote future success. Immediate, here-and-now interests and planning dominate in the short-term orientation.

Although relatively independent of one another, these dimensions do have connections between themselves, as well as with other possible axes and factors. Traditional cultures are usually masculine, have high levels of uncertainty avoidance and power distance, are collectivistic, and have short-term orientation, while modern ones usually feature femininity, low levels of uncertainty avoidance and power distance, individualism, and long-term orientation. Such a formal and generalized reference point, naturally, has quite a few exclusions. Traditional cultures of the East, for instance, as a rule have long-term orientations: this is in concordance with the Confucian aphorism that he who does not look far ahead must soon expect troubles. In general, the Confucian dimension is more applicable to Eastern cultures.

Wealthy cultures are individualistic, democratic, rational, less religious, and less obsessed with the idea of survival. *Poverty culture*[43] is characterized not so much by material poorness, but by the view of limited welfare, according to which gaining wealth is only possible at the expense of others. This view is related to deducible theories of equality, suspicion of the wealthy and successful people, disbelief that success is achievable through hard work, and refusal of long-term planning. Through these traits, poverty culture approximates Hofstede's short-term orientation. The Bulgarian cultural anthropologist M. Minkov, a follower of Hofstede's, supplements his dimensions with hypometropia (*short sightedness*), industry vs. indulgence, and monumentalism (associated with national dignity and a cult of the forefathers).[143] The high index of hypometropia, for instance, in Africa, Latin America, and many ghettos, is associated with high frequencies of murder, HIV, and pregnancy in adolescence.

Other dimensions are the religious vs. secular approach and values of survival vs. values of expression. A study by the World Bank demonstrates that gross domestic product is parallel to the secular approach and values of expression, and increases along with these dimensions.[223] The culture of Western, educated, industrialized, rich, and democratic countries is sometimes denoted by the acronym WEIRD, as if to suggest its strangeness, and to indicate that it represents a small sample of mankind—a cultural exclusion, rather than the rule.

The IC index is related to expressed emotions,[138] care for the elderly and babies, and disease. The relationship between culture and disease is a strong one—infectious and joint diseases, malnutrition, and chronic diarrhea proliferate in collectivistic communities, with diabetes, hypertension, and oncological disorders being more common in individualistic ones. Diabetes and hypertension are, as a rule, rare in traditional communities; however, they can be particularly common and severe among some members who are rapidly westernized, e.g., among urban Arabs or in the Tanzanian Hadza tribe. The relationship between this index and cardio-vascular diseases, as well as the so-called type A behavior (a Western culture specific syndrome, Chapter 11), is especially pronounced.[133] Social isolation causes increased mortality, while cultural dissonance between the individual and the community raises the prevalence of both physical and mental illnesses.

The distinction between high-contextual and low-contextual cultures is based on the degree to which behavior is influenced by the context: high in traditional, and low in modern cultures. Attitudes towards alcohol and sex are other possible dimensions for cultural assessment. Achievements in literature, philosophy, the arts, and technological progress, have been associated with cultures displaying sexual liberty[181] and tolerance to drinking since antiquity (Chapter 10). Furthermore, the national neuroticism dimension correlates with alcohol consumption, smoking, and suicides,[143] with France, Estonia, and Bulgaria leading in this regard.

Other possible cultural axes include attitudes to time and talking. In traditional communities, strict accounting for time and precise dating are not of as great importance as in modern ones. There, commonly, birthdays are not celebrated, and many people only know some approximation of their own age or that of their relatives. A good analogue to the English proverb "Time is money" is the Turkish saying "*Vaktim parasizdir*" (time does not cost money). The time measure of the twenty-four-hour period has over millennia been done in the way first put forth by the ancient people of the Middle East—with the start of the period at 6:00 AM instead of midnight. It is still measured in this way by some Arabs and in some African countries (as opposed to the official "English time"), and in Bulgaria, the transition from "Turkish" to "Frank" time symbolically marked a cultural pre-orientation, shortly followed by the country's liberation from Ottoman domination and the rise of the Third Bulgarian kingdom (1878). Beyond that, incessant chatter serves, in some traditional cultures as a kind of passive entertainment which also plays a defensive role in keeping the attention on constant alert.[47]

In collectivistic communities, the difference between in-group and between-group relationships is apparent; for individualistic communities, this line is less distinguishable. Physical attractiveness everywhere is associated not just with sex appeal, but also social skills, dominance, intelligence, and wealth, though notions about attractiveness vary. Heavier bodies are valued in Africa; in Japan—bigger eyes and smaller mouths. It is a rule that such distinctions are more readily recognized in people from the same group, and that others "all look alike". Love and intimacy do not play the same role in attraction, affairs, or marriage outside the cultures of Europe and North America; in many other places, marriages are still usually prearranged. Gender roles are based on stable stereotypes, although there are data related to personality structure on the so-called 5-factor model which demonstrate universal differences between men and women across cultures.[40, 133] For egalitarian societies like the Netherlands, these differences are smaller, while in traditional ones, such as Pakistan, they are more prominent. Conformity and submission are encouraged in many places, while in others (e.g., the United States) they are regarded as harmful and a hindrance to development. Meanwhile, large international corporations develop their own organizational cultures, requiring, first of all, a sense of belonging and the partial obliteration of one's cultural distinctions of origin.

Herodotus described how the Egyptians and Hellenes were different from each other,[220] and Julius Caesar and Tacitus described the Celts and Germans *through* the eyes of the Romans. The age of great geographical discoveries initiated descriptions of native cultures through the eyes of Europeans. The "global village" today has not brought about the homogenization which may have been expected and sometimes even reinforces cultural distinctions. Although used to emphasize its tolerance, the West is not always tolerant precisely when its liberal values are contested. There are universal values, though, such as liberty, and people from different cultures do similarly accept them—with the caveat that they do so for themselves, while differing in how far they are willing to accept these on behalf of others. People from poor countries, who travel rarely, consider their cultures to be superior over the cultures of the rest of the world, and, vice versa, those from rich countries do not agree: at the bottom of this ranking are Germany and the UK, and at the top are India, Bangladesh, and Pakistan.[143] As the understanding of other people's viewpoints is key to personal development, so does the knowledge of other cultures help in achieving a more sober outlook, the refusal of civilizational haughtiness, and acceptance of others. For at least two thirds of mankind, Lao Tzu, the Prophet Mohamed, Trotsky, or Che Guevara offer far more adequate explanatory matrices of the world than ever could Socrates, Hobbes, Montesquieu, or Hegel. And the appearance of new forms of identities,[157] or the development of a new world order and new civilizational rules, inevitably passes through the experience of feeling orphaned and having lost one's cultural roots (Chapter 13).

3 Cultural Context at Home: the Bulgarian Odysseus

> Troy is reachable; still unreachable is Ithaca.
>
> T. Zhechev

There hardly exists any Bulgarian who would not furrow their brow suspiciously at the idea of anyone attempting to summarize the Bulgarian mentality. But, then again, one would be hard pressed to find any French, Portuguese, or Maasai person who wouldn't react similarly when confronted with generalizations about their people. While stereotypes are readily accepted towards others, they seem to be only provisionally applied when it comes to ourselves (Chapter 2). Inside the community, individual variety is appreciated and labels—otherwise, easily attached to others—are rejected. The very notion of specific national qualities, or something resembling a national character, is extremely contestable[27, 76, 143] and misleading. Factor analysis of personality traits, for instance, demonstrates a universal personality structure,[133] while diversity of temperament and character is evident in all known human communities. The construct of a nation itself is a relatively new one (since the end of the 18th century), and is neither ethnically nor socially homogeneous. At the same time, particular communities' ethnic and cultural characteristics are well differentiated, and are clearly related to the manifestations of both mental health and illness (Chapter 5). Despite conceptual and political vagueness about what ethnicity means, it has been found that ethnic signs have a more pronounced impact on cultural traits and psychopathology than the influences of national affiliation, geographical proximity, historical ties, or religion.[115] Therefore, each exercise in national characterology should take ethnic priorities into consideration. Insight about our own cultural context and trends contributes not only to understanding illness in this context, but also to answering questions like why do we not succeed, why are we different,[143] or why has the Bulgarian Odysseus[225] not yet returned.

3.1 Antinomies of the Bulgarian Mentality

A basic feature of Bulgarian culture is its *intermediate* place between modern and traditional communities, along with the simultaneous presence of traits from these two cultural types, which results in diversity, transitional forms, and nuanced socio-psychological characteristics. For large strata of the population, these characteristics are close to those typical for modern culture, while for closed and nonintegrated communities, they are closer to the traditional pole. Traditional and modern lie at opposite ends of a continuum full of intermediates, where the *gradient* modern-traditional is in the direction heading from the ethnic Bulgarian population to the Gypsy and Turkish ethnic groups, from urban to rural, from well-educated to less educated, from the young to the elderly, and from the socially mobile to those living among extended kin. The communities comprised of Gypsies and Turks are themselves not homogeneous, but, in general, keep closer to traditional cultural signs than do Bulgarians. There are apparent deviations from this rule, especially for young and mobile people, among whom the cosmopolitan traits of youth culture dominate over traditional ethnic signs. The modern-traditional gradient can be traced in each of the following descriptive characteristics.

A *non-homogeneous identity* has been determined by the historical trajectory and rise of the Bulgarian people and state organization: not because of differentiation from others, but because of nomadic and settled ethnicities being united and assimilated. The nation's intermediate position between the traditional and the modern aspects of collective self-awareness comes from its concomitant belonging to both Europe and the Orient. Contradictory characterological clichés, such as gaiety and crudeness, industry and idleness, hospitality and suspicion, dignity and treachery, are expressions of the lack of homogeneous self-knowledge and identity splitting. As in one of the Roman dynasties, good and bad Claudii[72] are displayed—polar masks of the same family—most commonly fluctuating between insolence (usually towards those below us) and servility (usually towards those above us). Identity represents the degree of cohesion of images of self and others.[78] In the course of development, a mature identity with well consolidated images of self and others is preceded by a phase in which these images, though well discriminated, are parceled into good and bad parts.[112] *Marginal identity*—and its clinical analogue, borderline personality disorder—has become frozen in this phase of development, where contrasting aspects of self-images and those of others are kept in isolation by the defense mechanism of splitting, therein sparing the anxiety of complete self-knowledge and causing polarized notions. In social psychology, marginal personalities are sometimes described as those which possess varied social roles that spread across the borders of different realities—immigrants, priests, actors, psychiatrists, and educated women are given as examples.[187] They are said to be more labile, but also more creative.

One of the consequences of such splitting is the experience of unpredictability, manifested through *fatalism*—the view that life depends on forces beyond one's control.[43] Its product is the behavior of *learnt helplessness*, with its characteristic cultural clichés like "chance", "being born in the wrong place and at the wrong time", or "it's out of my hands". A fatalistic view of life is incidental to cultures of *poverty*, where the idea of limited welfare instills the notion that one person's prosperity can only come at the expense of others (Chapter 2). In these cultures, there is pressure not to stand out coupled with envy towards successful individuals, as well as respect for seniority, personal connections, and external signs of wealth and status. Contrary to a strong work ethic, a poverty mentality is dominated by the attitude that effort is undeserved and planning is unnecessary.[43] This lack of perspective is close to Hofstede's short-term orientation,[87] and Minkov's hypometropia (short-sightedness)[143]. This splitting is also displayed in a certain affinity for dualistic heresies: from Manichaeism and the influential Bogomils—a movement named after Bogomil the Priest which spread from the Balkans up to Languedoc in Southwestern France in the Middle Ages—to embraced theories of class struggle and antagonism towards the establishment, unending partisan bipolarity, and eclectic antipodes of art and taste.

The *patriarchal spirit* is vividly illustrated in E. Berne's book *Games People Play*,[19] where, among typical archetypal situations (*games*) presented in the paradigm of transactional analysis, the prototype of the *peasant* is described. This a Bulgarian peasant woman with arthritis who sells her only cow in order to afford treatment at a university clinic in Sofia. The professor uses her as an interesting case to make clinical demonstrations to an audience of students, causing her admiration at his frequent use of Latin terms. Discharged without any improvement, she receives a prescription and treatment instructions which she cannot fulfill due to the lack of conditions necessary for hydrotherapy and dieting in her village (and as far as the prescription is concerned, she would never part with this valuable piece of paper). Despite this, she frequently tells stories about the great professor, and prays for him. Years later, the professor passes through her village, while visiting a rich and demanding private patient, and as she recognizes him, she rushes to kiss his hand, blessing him for the marvelous treatment. Flattered, he fails to notice that her joints are more deformed than before.

One of the manifestations of this characteristic is the strong influence of family in making decisions related to illness. In a long-term follow up of Bulgarian patients with schizophrenia, we found that the burden of the disease is carried, above all, by the family—a peculiar substitute for care services[67, 68] (Chapter 8). In a study on melancholia among Bulgarians, Kirov[116] points out that delusions of guilt during psychotic depression are directed most commonly towards the family, more often than when compared to other populations where such moral stances are taken in relationship to God or the fatherland. The role of the family or clan is particularly apparent in group pressure for involuntary treatment (Chapter 12), sometimes including "tribal jail" for deviants. In rural populations and among ethnic minority groups, the family offers a group alliance, one that ensures basic confidence in never being abandoned. The more isolated a community is, the more powerful the role of the clan, and the more unfeasible informed consent and individual choice, become.

Sexist traits are a separate aspect of the patriarchal mentality. Although in some closed communities they are expressed to the extent of male chauvinism, in the larger part of contemporary Bulgarian society they have been left to history. Values, role models and expectations, however, do not die out so rapidly. Power, strength, the ability to make money and impose order, physical might, and wit are all highly valued qualities that are unambiguously associated with masculinity. The consequences of these traits are the acceptance of psychological suffering as a weakness, and a higher threshold for recognizing and enduring problems, and hence, for searching for mental help in men than in women. The expectations of the roles of adolescents also determine the degree of their behaviors' pathologization: the same behavior may be bad for a boy and sick for a girl. Sexist cultural sanctions can phenomenologically display similar temperamental labilities in men and women, by different means.[136] And yet, cultural attitudes of submissiveness on the part of the female role finds their specific display in the pathological family dynamics of alcoholics' families.

Materialism may be most succinctly characterized by an expression coined by the inimitable revolutionary and chronicler Dzhendo (aka Zahari Stoyanov), that every liberty is lethal to the Bulgarian if it is not tied to the home, goods, cornfields, vineyards, and mature wormwood wine.[199] Religiosity has never been profound among Bulgarians; Turks still linger far from a strict adherence to Islamic canons; and Gypsies commonly use it as an ad hoc means of adjustment. Since the days of Christian conversion (9th century), the Orthodox Church has bred resistance and heresy,[193] while pagan ritualism and symbolism have preserved their great diversity.[12, 213] The conundrums "The ox yelled in a deep ravine, the foxes heard him and waved their tails" or "the priest started singing, the women crossed themselves" hold no particular sacrality. The combination of materialistic values with the lack of a steady transcendent mainstay, and a relative shortage of material welfare, causes deprivation. The absence of pronounced religiosity is partially substituted by superstitions[17] and affinities for magical cures. Stories of magic do not bear transcendent signs, but are rather pagan, utilitarian, and commonplace. Some magical rituals are analogous to psychopathological phenomena. The link between the first person entering the house on *Ignajden* (December 20), called the *polaznik*, and the home's fate during the new year, is a model of obsession. The imitative and contagious mechanisms of magic (Chapter 6) can be traced in the *koledari, survakari, kukeri* (whose authentic versions always feature the rite of touching with a wooden phallus), *rusalii, nestinari* (Chapter 7), *lazaruvane*, the act of asking for forgiveness, sorcery, casting spells, and the rich symbolic pantomimes of many holidays, such as *Todorovden* (St. Todor's day), when, for instance, women neigh like mares and kick each other so that they may give birth to "colts".[12]

Consideration of *brains*, at the expense of emotions, is deeply embedded in Bulgarian culture, and commonly manifests itself in the traditional respect towards education, along with steadfast dedication and sacrifices made in order to ensure it for one's children. An instrumental and practically oriented intellect is valued, as opposed to abstract reasonings, e.g., philosophy, and their occupation. Utilitarian instructions, and not cosmogonic theories, are expected from religions as a rule. This respect for intellect contrasts with a negligence of the emotional side of psychic life, to the extent that the display of feelings is identified with weakness. Bulgarians are sometimes characterized by others as knowledgeable, but having no refined instincts[76]—a dissociation between brains and barbarity, something probably intrinsic to all Balkan populations. In clinical practice, caring for relatives is much more adequate with regard to taking medicine, the material environment, and guardedness, than it is with regard to the emotional needs of the patient.

One of the consequences of this pragmatic orientation is *cultural anhedonia*. Balkan cultures are traditionally described as rough.[12, 76, 177, 213, 225] Overt displays of feelings, especially tender ones, are not encouraged. A symbolic manifestation of this trait is the centuries-old regional custom of very tightly fastening babies' diapers. It is also anecdotally reflected in the saying that, while elsewhere children usually sleep like angels, in the Balkans they sleep as though being slaughtered, as well as in the proverb, "If your guts are trailing on the ground, say that your belt has unrolled". This cold-bloodedness and stoicism create an atmosphere of taboos, repressed spontaneity, emotional self-awareness, personal sharing, and impulsiveness; the clinical manifestation of distress is channeled not through feelings, but through alcohol sedation and violent outbursts, particularly in men.[155]

In Hofstede's cultural dimensions,[87] this culture can be characterized by masculinity, high degrees of uncertainty avoidance and power distance, and collectivistic and short-term orientations, as well as the hypometropia and monumentalism of Minkov's dimensions,[143] with the stipulation that for each

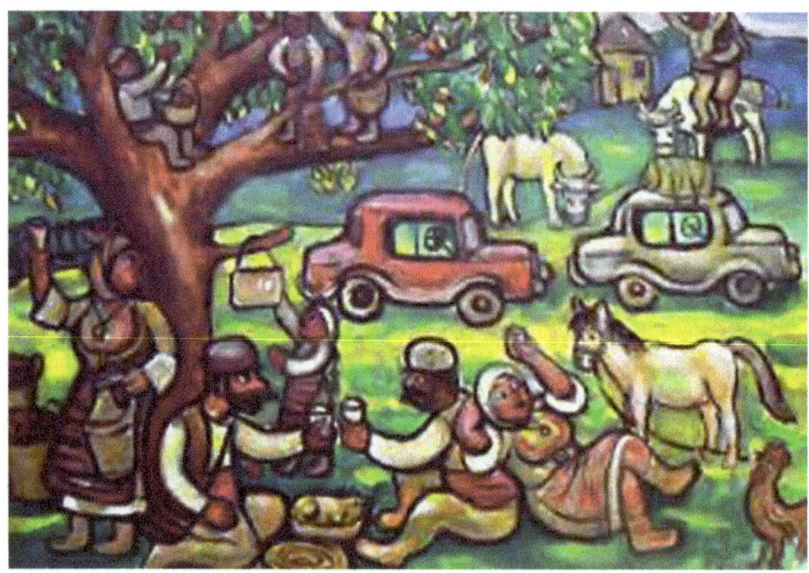

Fig. 1: Bulgarians, painting by Stoyan Venev

of these, the modern-traditional gradient maintains polarity between urbanized and closed communities, the educated and the uneducated, and Bulgarians and minorities. Additionally, a World Bank study on orientation and values shows[223] that Bulgarian culture is closer to a secular orientation than a religious one, and it shares more of the values of survival than it does those of expression.

Steady cultural characteristics are shaken in times of change, thus causing *de-culturation*: the loss of cultural mainstays, with new cultural rules not yet acquired. This is the major phenomenon which marks the experience of rapid change, and has domineered contemporary Bulgarian culture for decades. Its beginning was back in the 50s and the 60s of the 20th century, with mass urbanization, industrialization, people being ripped away from their peasant roots, and the forceful establishment of a working-class culture in panel-block ghettoes. Nostalgia for the old patriarchal spirit, expressed by P.R. Slaveikov, the poet who fought for Bulgaria's church autonomy in the 1860s, was used a century later by an influential literary critic as a metaphor for the socialist uprooting.[225] No culture is pathogenic in itself. However, rapid cultural change, and especially from traditional to modern values, has pathogenic potential in specific ways: through cultural identity confusion—the conflict between traditional and imported values; through anomia—the breakdown of social bonds and loss of old cultural rules governing behavior; and through deprivation—the experience of privation and being underprivileged due to the gap between a newly sought-after way of life and economic reality.[183] Identity is more homogeneous in ethnic minorities, but their mobile layers are more threatened by the effects of cultural change, because the distance between their traditional core and modernity, hurriedly acquired, is larger. In their identity, they are *cultural nomads*. Clinical manifestations of cultural change include rising rates of alcoholism, drug addiction, and suicide.

Since basic cultural rules are unconscious and unwritten (Chapter 2), good cultural integration assumes that one does not contemplate over them, e.g., the manner of salutation or gestures. Cultural change is dramatized precisely when the unwritten rules are questioned. An indicator of such dramatization is *heightened self-introspection*: what are we? Why are we what we are? Similarly, healthy individuals do not monitor their own automatized experiences; on the other hand, excessively focusing on them, combined with losing the sense of their natural datum, may be a clinical symptom. Thus, increased interest and a tendency towards analyzing community functioning may indicate cultural alienation. Besides its pathogenic role, the main cultural transition in the country—from a fatalistic mentality to personal autonomy—also contains huge potential for development, yet this remains unrecognized due to the blindness caused by a traumatic view of life.

3.2 Traumatic Memory and an "Optimistic Theory"

Self-experience in Bulgarian culture is traumatic. As in individual post-traumatic stress disorder, the collective memory is saturated with reproductions of tragic events from the past, and the current functioning is dominated by the avoidance of nightmares and signs of losses and self-destructive behaviors, such as drunkenness and suicidal driving. Negative self-assessment, complaining, and self-negation are considered by many[12, 57, 77, 116, 225] to be the leading traits of the national mentality. Their cultural roots are embedded in collective memory, which is selectively obsessed with historical and geographical misfortunes, losses, victims, betrayals, mean neighbors, and the Great Powers, and constant failure. Pessimism, the "spirit of negation", or "Bulgarian melancholy"[57] embrace all aspects of life, not only the past, although their origin is in the past, sometimes traced back to the destructive passions of the proto-Bulgarians, relatives of the Huns. Remembering is a moral imperative; however, the matter of what is worth remembering is a cultural choice—and it is certainly a choice of identity. Much like the unabolished memory of the Holocaust forms the basis of modern

European identity,[108] the memory of (real or imaginary) failures marks contemporary Bulgarian identity.

At a personal level, this identity operates, again, through denial: I am an exclusion to this—the idiom "the Bulgarian way" refers to *others*. Such identification through discrimination causes negative stereotypes towards one's own cultural origin, along with a compensatory inflated self-image, or leads to a new antinomy: extreme individualism, albeit within a patriarchal culture. The contemporary Bulgarian traumatic mentality is, above all things, a narcissistic wound of anti-utopian nationalism. It is a cultural phenomenon, not as a result of the ontological past, but because of its interpretation. The national ideal—in the form shaped by the ideological dreams of Rakovski during the Bulgarian Renaissance, the geographical map of the San Stefano draft treaty for national liberation (1878), and the apologists of the Balkan Wars at the beginning of the 19th century—remains unfulfilled, and this unfulfillment is so blinding that it does not allow for lessons to be drawn from history. The ambition to realize this ideal form, one that has caused national catastrophes, sustained by unlearnt lessons, is tragically predestined like in an Ancient Greek tragedy, as if replaying the fallacy of Croesus. According to Herodotus, the Delphi oracle prophesied that Croesus would destroy a large kingdom, if he started a war against the Persian King Cyrus. He started one, and the prophecy came true—he destroyed his own kingdom.[220]

The traumatic view of life operates as a cultural filter by selectively sifting out and exaggerating negative aspects, thus missing the grounds for a truly "optimistic theory" (I. Hadjiisky)[77] about our own people. This blindness is supported by its counter-arguments. Negative self-assessments need compensation for reasons of pride, which—like negative self-assessment itself—is plainly groundless next to countrified self-vaunting. False self-assessments, in a self-defensive manner, refuse to recognize the real problems in collective history, replacing them instead with traumatic memories. Thereby, a double blindness about self-knowledge is achieved—the failure to distinguish what is really valuable from the gloomy reading of collective fortune results in compensatory self-aggrandizing through proxies and whitewashing real problems. For this reason, playing the part of *victims* hinders the acknowledgment and admittance of the exterminations, or other documented atrocities, that *we* have caused to others such as Pomaks, Turks, and Greeks.

Cognitive distortions about the positive aspects of self-assessment and historical trajectory follow all of its vicissitudes. Tragic memories about foreign occupations (i.e., Byzantine and Ottoman), adhering to them the label of slavery, do not admit the facts that the country was, throughout these periods, among the most prosperous and desirable provinces to live in of at least three world empires. Since the Roman Empire, the land's mineral springs have been a favorite destination of the aristocracy on their holidays, and its status as a privileged province for centuries preserved the language, religion, and ethnic composition, also allowing crafts and trade to develop. Serdika (today's Sofia) was the emperor's residence when, in 311 CE, the Edict of Toleration by Galerius was issued there, thus legalizing Christianity—probably the most significant political act from the period of antiquity and its transition to the Middle Ages.

Peering back at losses and the deprivation of territories does not allow for the acknowledgment of the old Bulgarians' predatory state ambitions, as they created states through the establishment of military encampments on their path from Asia to Europe, with the Balkan version being the oldest national state in Europe to have kept the same name, over a period which lasted for 13 centuries. Just a few years after the settlement of Asparukh's Bulgarians in the Northeastern part of the Balkan peninsula, a well-functioning customs office was already in operation—epitomizing a state structure with efficient institutions. These ambitions of expansion also played a strong separatist role, especially during the Second Bulgarian kingdom, which had, during the major part of its existence, only conditional centralized power—but this was true of most European states at that time. Self-defamation does not recognize the mission of these militaristic, arrogant, and "unclean" (in Byzantine terms) people as cultural carriers: the Bulgarian golden treasures from Nagy Szent Miklós and Mala Pereshchepina bear the exquisiteness of Iranian stylistics, and the monumental architecture at Pliska, Drustar, and Preslav (the largest and most thriving city in Eastern Europe after Constantinople during the early Middle Ages)[177] partially resembles not only Roman models but also the palaces of the Umayyad Caliphate.

Like the initially inefficient but militarized Scandinavian civilization, which flourished only after the spiritual inculcation of the Christian West even though vast territories of Christianity had been raided by the victorious Vikings,[207] so too were the ferocious Bulgarians, believing themselves to be descendants of the mythical Avitohol, inspired by their main enemy, the Eastern Roman Empire, to embrace Christianity and the Cyrillic alphabet, thus turning their civilization into a cradle of Slavonic-speaking Orthodox culture. But, in accordance with the tragic antinomies of national trajectory—the decay of the same Orthodox civilization was initiated by the 40-year bloody war with Byzantium at the end of the 9th and beginning of the 10th century.[206]

The most *archaic trauma* of collective memory is probably the slaughter of 52 noble *boila* clans during the conversion to Christianity in the 9th century. It marked with tragic feeling a turning point in the nation's fate, comparable to the massacre of the innocents by the order of King Herod—without, however, realizing the civilizational role of the new religion, in contrast with the evangelistic delight which came from the survival of the child Jesus in the land of Israel, soaked in blood. The cult of suffering denies that peace or security existed between the 15th and 17th centuries,[123] when roughly half of Europe's population was exterminated by wars and plague epidemics. It also denies the subsequent development of crafts—the proud guild mentality having nothing to do with the falsely alleged "slave psyche"[77]—as well as schools, religious autonomy, and the unique cultural institution of *chitalishtes*, community centers with libraries, amateur theaters, and discussion clubs.

The obsession with treachery does not recognize the gesture made by one Hadji Stanyo Vrabevski, a respected wealthy merchant from Teteven whose appearance in the *konaks* (Ottoman city councils) of Sofia and other large cities was met by the *kaymakamins* (Ottoman regional governors) standing up—the Hadji, having been sentenced for subversive activity and exiled in Diyarbakir, upon his return delivered to the new Bulgarian state authorities the cash he had been keeping for a secret committee. The rapt denigration of any kind of power or political partisanship fails to identify the real giants of the Bulgarian Renaissance and architects of contemporary Bulgaria[71] (replacing them with Russian counts and generals), especially those, such as Z. Stoyanov and S. Stambolov, who were able to self-educate themselves en route from illiteracy to the cosmopolitan confidence of visionaries. Disgracing the political class is a centuries-old tradition of alienating one's self from the state, beginning more than likely with the Adamite and Bogomil heretic movements during the Middle Ages. Clearly evident of this is the fact that such a rich folklore lacks many songs about tsars and boyars[77], with the only probable exception being one dedicated to Tsar Ivan Shishman, precisely the monarch who bowed down to Sultan Murad and put an end to the Second Bulgarian kingdom—again, a peculiar apotheosis of tragedy.

This attitude of envious proletarian degradation does not admit to the constructive impulses of the early 20th century or the brilliant, independent, and broad-minded personalities among the intellectual and political elites of that epoch;[225] neither is the fact that during World War II, Bulgaria was the only country in Europe[108] to have gained and not lost territory, without fighting, remembered—and all that while being on the wrong side of the powers. Self-humiliation as the most loyal Soviet satellite blinds the memory of the *Goryani* guerrillas, the most powerful anti-communist illegal movement in all of Eastern Europe in the 1950s. And the demonization of the transition following the collapse of totalitarianism cannot swallow the three-fold increase of gross domestic product at that time, which has no parallel in the country's history. Bulgaria's membership in the world's most elite clubs contradicts its simultaneous ranking—in unison with the traumatic mentality—as one of the worldwide leaders on the unhappiness index. This self-humiliation complex is seemingly ashamed of the inexhaustible cultural wealth of aphorisms, songs, riddles, games, erotic ritualism, magical worlds of traditional healers, goblins, stalkers, strange fairies, elves, sorcerers, the exotic subcultures of *kapantsi*, Gagauz, *karakachani*, and *kizilbashi*, not to mention a language that never fails to be colorful and is full of dialects, and even separate secret languages used by closed groups.

Cultural self-knowledge is a choice of viewpoint, not of facts. When choosing a pessimistic position, the facts do not matter. Being blind to the positive qualities of belonging and aspects of the past stabilizes a traumatic view of life and reproduces the behaviors of learnt helplessness, fatalism, and hopelessness. They choke out the energy for constructivism and soak into a masochistic daze, fed by the ceaseless whimpering of the victim. Scotoma surrounding the positive are toxic to self-awareness and motivation and, through a self-fulfilling prophecy, push towards national ruin. Insecurity about such self-awareness is so pronounced that the frequent use of the word "normal" as a synonym for things going smoothly has transformed it into an allegory of lethargy: normalcy is when nothing happens or changes. Cultural blindness does not allow for adequate lessons to be learnt, nor for us to move forward with confidence, while the self-underestimation it causes is compensated with vulgar showing off. One of the keenest thoughts about our self-knowledge was penned by the national hero V. Levski in one of his letters, referring to a serial Russian spy in the secret liberation network: "We have all been burned, and yet we do not know to blow on the tea". In these conditions of de-culturation, the victims' experience is dramatized and the pathogenic dimensions of de-culturation are overestimated, while its potential for development remains unrecognized due to the cultural *shortsightedness* of the traumatic view of life. Cultural transition, especially when preceded by cultural sedation, is confusing in its absence of rules but also contains a strong creative embryo, eloquently illustrated by some ages whose signs of resurgence have only been realized later on (Chapter 13). Overcoming negative thinking and self-pity is the only feasible way towards an "optimistic theory". Besides this, the only chance the Bulgarian Odysseus[225] has is to step out of his captivity, constructed by false notions about himself, and return to authenticity.

4 Psychopathology: Essence and Manifestation

> Individuality is the world as her own.
>
> G. Hegel

Psychopathology refers to both teaching about mental illness in general, and the entity of manifestations which may signify mental illness or psychological distress. In essence, these manifestations are experiences and behaviors. Symptoms of psychopathology occur, in fact, *experientially*, while motor and behavioral manifestations are its external expressions—also serving as the only outer markers of abnormal experience accessible for observation, as markers like laboratory findings or physical signs are lacking. Regardless of innumerable didactic descriptions, misunderstandings about psychopathology, even among professionals, generally arise from the notion that it represents some ontological reality with material signs. Since antiquity, a given phenomenon has usually denoted the appearance of things, as contrasted to their underlying meaning (lathomenon).[10] In the phenomenology of Heidegger, Husserl, and Jaspers, however, the term phenomenon is used for an inner, subjective experience. Jaspers[104] (Fig. 2) defines the experience as a *phenomenon* of the psyche, its genuine "objective fact", and not as the subjective shadow of another objectively observable occurrence. In contemporary psychiatry, there is instead a risk of new reductionism with attempts to reduce psychopathological phenomena to the biochemical level, neglecting their experiential aspect. The problem with epistemology in psychopathology stems from the objective-subjective rationale from the 19th-century positivist approach to the natural sciences being applied to the psyche. In psychopathology, experience is the objective phenomenon, while the position of the clinician assessing it remains subjective.

The phenomena of psychopathology change—in different ways, according to the syndrome and individual peculiarities—one's attitudes towards self and the world, thus creating an inner picture of the disease which does not coincide with the ontological reality of the observer. Rather, this constitutes a "world of one's own" with personal *signatura rerum* (signs of things)[104] coming from the morbid reflection of this reality. Individually altered attitudes towards self and/or the environment are the key to understanding psychopathology. Other characteristics

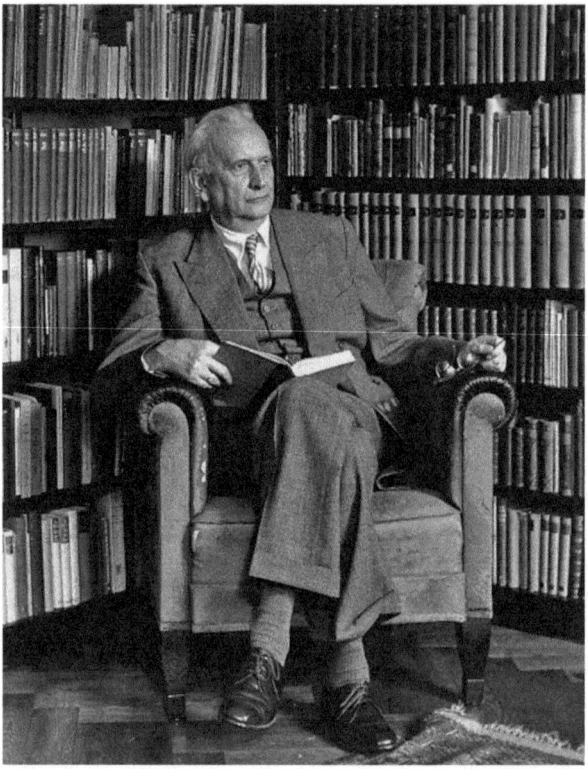

Fig. 2: Karl Jaspers (1883–1969) (Courtesy to Getty Images)

are the *quantitative deviation* of most symptoms from their normal analogues; and the *deterioration of functioning*. These, and not the symptom content, discriminate symptom from normal experience. A normal prototype, e.g., sadness for depression, or shyness for anxiety, transforms into a symptom, when it meets certain quantitative criteria (in terms of frequency, intensity, or duration) which disturb habitual individual functioning. The specific quantitative criteria are determined by field trials in the general population, usually during the preparation of new editions to international classifications. The symptoms' content may be extremely out of the ordinary; however, if quantitative differences and dysfunction are missing, no symptom exists. Another common criterion, subjective distress, is not obligatory and may be absent, as in mania, paraphrenias, personality pathologies, or addictions.

4.1 The Syndrome

General psychopathology recognizes and describes pathological mental manifestations, organizing them into areas and levels of impairment, presented commonly by mental domains or syndromes. The assessment of different *domains* of the psyche include the following symptom groups:

Psychomotorics—unlike neurological motor disturbances which have no experiential correlates, here changes in posture and motor behavior which reflect the inner state, are included: mimicry through expressions of, for example, sadness, fright, or indifference; retardation to immobility and stupor, or agitation; and catatonic phenomena like stupor, excitement, freezing into poses, stereotypical movements, waxy flexibility, echolalia, or echopraxia.

Consciousness—quantitative alteration of one's clarity of consciousness (level of alertness or vigilance): ranging from mental cloudiness to coma; or qualitative alteration with sensory impairment and loss of orientation to time, space, or self, leading to confusion.

Perceptions—abnormal perceptions distorting a real object (illusions), or presenting a non-existent one (hallucinations): according to the affected sense modality, they may be auditory, visual, olfactory, gustatory, tactile, or vestibular.

Attention—the degree of focusing, with disturbances (hypoprosexia) either in its active (poor concentration), or passive (distractibility) aspect.

Emotions—the lasting emotional background (mood) and the outwardly displayed emotional response (affect), which color the total attitude to reality: low mood (dysthymia), infectious (hyperthymia) or silly (euphoria) elevation, a constricted emotional range (affective flattening), indifference (apathia), anger (dysphoria), or inappropriate emotional responses (parathymia), as well as their intensity, duration, lability, and control.

Will—the energy needed for purposeful activity, including choice of aim, struggle between motives and contra-motives, and decision making and execution: it may be decreased (hypoboulia), excessive (hyperboulia), or qualitatively deformed (paraboulia).

Thinking—the cognitive instrument for realizing intellectual potential and whose disturbances may affect: speed of thought processes, e.g., accelerated or retarded; form of thought, e.g., circumstantial, neological, paralogical, incoherent; or content of thought, e.g., overvalued ideas, obsessions, or delusions.

Memory—cognitive function for preserving and reproducing information which, depending on how far the event lies in the past, can be immediate (seconds to minutes), short-term (several days), or long-term (remote past), while its loss (amnesia) may affect: different stages of the process which include the fixation, retention, and reproduction of remembered material; or different periods in relation to the moment of impairment—before (retrograde), during (congrade), or after (anterograde) it. Other disturbances are distortions of memories, and filling in memory gaps with unreal stories (confabulation).

Intellect—the cognitive potential which is realized through thinking, and factors into the discovery of correlations, problem solving, and mastering of abstractions: its impairment can be inborn (mental retardation) or acquired (dementia).

In the format of such separate assessments across different domains, general psychopathology tends to estimate higher cortex functions rather than psychopathological entities. In thought disorders, for instance, impairments in executive functions which closely mirror the mechanisms of short-term memory and attention, are obvious; but despite this, formal thought disorders are traditionally associated with disturbances of thought structure, not memory or attention disturbances. In clinical reality, the phenomena cluster in *syndromes*. These are not casual, mechanical sums of symptoms, but form coherent pictures of manifestations that appear to be understandable in a clinical context, e.g., depressive thinking accompanied by low drives and emotions in depressive syndrome. The syndrome reflects "the momentary wholeness"[104] of the inner picture of illness. For this reason, psychopathology is syndromology, not symptomatology. Its focus on the leading syndrome—and not on separate clinical fragments—in the diagnostic process, transforms it, to paraphrase Jablensky, into an *antidote* to spurious comorbidity.[97] Most psychiatric diagnoses do not meet the criteria of nosological entities, and are, in fact, syndromes, e.g., depression. Furthermore, out of all the psychopathological domains, consciousness and psychomotorics ensure the most efficient vision into the core of the syndrome—consciousness, by ensuring access to other domains of assessment; and motor disturbances, as a direct nonverbal demonstration of drive and emotional impairment. Both also influence every other manifestation, many of which may be inaccessible to assessment during a severe episode.

Despite its wealth of clinical pictures and individual diversity, psychopathology is manifested through combinations and variations of a *limited* number of basic syndromes. Like all organs, the brain has a limited set of homeostatically and evolutionarily sustained reactions which manifest themselves automatically, thus saving energy for specific creations by each pathogenic agent, for more adaptive purposes. Clinical variety can be reduced to variants and combinations of these basic syndromes. The order of their presentation, from anxious to organic ones, follows the rise of their relative specificity and role in the diagnostic hierarchy. Anxiety syndromes are the most unspecific, and hierarchically take up the lowest diagnostic rank, while organic syndromes are more specific, ranking in hierarchical priority over others in diagnostic respects.

Anxiety

Anxiety is a universal human reaction to insecurity and threat. When it is excessive and does not correspond with a reason, it may reach pathological proportions and impede daily functioning—manifesting itself, generally, into three groups of symptoms: mental, e.g., excessive worrying, apprehension, and fear; muscular, e.g., the inability to relax and achiness; and autonomous, i.e., sympathetic excitement (palpitation, mouth dryness, sweating, gut motility, and dizziness).

As a syndrome, anxiety is *unspecific*, frequently accompanies many physical and mental diseases, and may be a sign of abnormal illness behavior. Only when not present with another disease, excessive anxiety is at the basis of anxiety disorders. Regardless of specific manifestations in the different forms of anxiety disorders, e.g., panic disorder or agoraphobia, the common characteristics are irrational fears, excessive autonomous reactivity, tension, and fainting with anticipation of physical collapse. Somatization and dissociation, with their vast cultural diversity, are frequent masks of anxiety (Chapter 9).

Depression

Depression is a syndrome characterized by lasting low mood, inability to experience pleasure (anhedonia), loss of energy, weight, sleep, appetite, or libido, motor retardation, uneasiness and agitation, low self-esteem or feelings of guilt, retarded thinking, poor concentration, difficulty making decisions, and thoughts of death or suicide. Normal prototypes of these manifestations are quite well known. Clinical depression, however, is not a trivial experience; on the contrary, it is stable and not influenced by external stimuli, and it also profoundly affects the ability to cope with daily life. Low mood has different nuances: sad, dull, despondent, indifferent, empty, desperate. The syndrome has various forms depending on combinations of the described manifestations. Although there is some agreement that low mood and impairment of the ability to experience pleasure should always be present, this does not refer to all cultures (Chapter 9).

Depressively colored thinking is, as a rule, retarded, monotonous, and filled with fruitlessness or bluntness, and thought content shows congruence with emotions: ideas of incompetence, failure, loss of meaning, poverty, lack of perspective, and exaggeration of faults and guilt. Sleep is usually disturbed in its later phase, with characteristic early awakening, and the overall experience is more painful in the morning. Lowered drives can cause refusal to eat, weight loss, the neglect of hygiene, and severe immobility (depressive stupor). Combined with anxiety, it results in marked uneasiness, to the extent of agitation, the inability to stay still, noisy breathing and sighing, and aimless fidgeting. In some atypical forms, there may be excessive eating (without, however, experiencing pleasure from food), weight gain, and sleepiness. The main risk in depression is of suicide. Severe depression may be complicated by psychotic symptoms, most commonly delusions of guilt (i.e., psychotic depression). Depression lacks a high level of specificity, and although it is a basic syndrome of the affective disorders, it may also occur in the course of almost all mental disorders.

Mania

Mania is a syndrome marked by increased drives and levels of vigilance and activity, manifesting with: permanently heightened (hyperthymia) or irritable moods; increased initiatives and activity; decreased tiredness and need for sleep; pressure of speech; accelerated mental activity—to the extent of flight of ideas and extreme distractibility; increased self-evaluation—to the extent of megalomaniac delusion; increased libido and familiarity; and decreased insight.

Sometimes manic patients are viewed by others not as mentally ill, but rather as arrogant or intoxicated. The milder form of the syndrome (hypomania) may, in fact, provide some selective advantage with increased sociability, libido, and energy. Full-blown manic syndrome, however, can hardly go unrecognized. Heightened emotionality is not concordant with external events, and may manifest itself as either contagious and fun, or with anger (dysphoria). This behavior is dominated by expressive motorics, excessive spending, unreasonable initiatives, increased sexuality, talkativeness (frequently with a hoarse voice), distractibility, grandiose posturing, and a manner of powerfulness.

Thinking and speech are accelerated, with rapid shifts between topics, sometimes achieved via associations with rhymes and puns, or with expansive ideas about the content: from unrealistic self-overvaluation to megalomaniac delusions (of wealth, talent, celebrity, noble descent, etc.) in psychotic mania. When the syndrome is severe, it may present alongside excitement, unintelligible speech, and dangerous behavior (confused mania). Mania is the basic syndrome of bipolar affective disorder.

Acute psychosis

Psychosis is a broad concept, applied to a large group of syndromes with altered (as compared to individual and culturally normalized) attitudes towards reality, incorrigibility, and the presence of symptoms such as delusions, hallucinations, or disorganized behavior. Acuteness is a term denoting both abruptness in onset (in terms of days), and the pattern of symptom manifestation—stormy, emotionally intense, and unsteady. The signs of acuteness are: delusional mood, disturbance in motor behavior, and sleeplessness. The more acute the state, the more pronounced these signs become. They are obligatory, unlike more specific psychotic symptoms like delusions and hallucinations, which may be absent or only apparent later on. The basic symptom of the syndrome is a delusional mood, or delusional affect, usually accompanied by delusional perceptions. A delusional mood is the sudden inrush of powerful experiences of bewilderment, puzzlement, or enlightenment; or the suddenly and painfully clear revelation of one's vision about things, including the covert deciphering of the meanings behind an otherwise visibly unaltered environment—these are frequently enigmatic or frightening. As a rule, this symptom precedes the formation of delusions. The delusional mood is viewed by Jaspers[104] as a model of alterations made to the internal picture of the world, and, when dominated by ecstasy, it resembles the mystical states of some religious cults (Chapter 6).

Besides these basic signs, at the onset of the psychotic episode there are also frequently non-specific complaints, withdrawal, or staring present. They are followed by rapid escalation, with intense, usually fearful, affect, and symptoms indicative of psychosis:

- hallucinations—such as hearing voices, or sensing strange smells or tastes; or delusional perceptions—wrong interpretivisms with otherwise intact perceptions, e.g., receiving special messages from real objects;
- delusions—incorrigible ideas that frequently develop as explanations for other unusual experiences with emotional intensity, not allowing for alternatives (e.g., mere chance) and including such convictions as the idea that one's thoughts are being recorded, that one is being poisoned, followed, or watched, or is the victim of experimentation;
- so-called first-rank symptoms of schizophrenia—characterized by experiences of external intrusions into one's mental activities and loss of control over them, e.g., feeling as though being revealed, speaking thoughts aloud, thought broadcasting, thought insertion, thought blocking, thought withdrawal (frequently interpreted as thoughts being stolen), and the replacement of one's volition, emotions and thoughts with alien ones;

- catatonic symptoms—such as freezing in poses, catalepsy with waxy flexibility, stereotypies, imitative acts, or chaotic destructiveness;
- disorganized and impulsive behavior;
- formal thought disorder—such as unclear, or tangential speech, peculiar turns of phrase, metonymies, neologisms, and incoherence, to the extent of "word salad" and complete unintelligibility.

These psychotic symptoms change the individual's behavior, sometimes beyond recognition, and directly control it. The psychotic individual may take measures for self-defense, accuse, warn others about an imminent threat, or transmit coded messages to and from "chasers" or "rescuers". Their contact with reality is interrupted, cutting off accessibility of correction through evidence or by reasons of logic and common sense. The fact that one's views are not shared by others, instead of shaking such opinions, frequently rather increases certainty that a plot exists. Depending on the prevailing symptoms, the acute psychotic syndrome may be cycloid, delusional, hallucinatory, delusional-hallucinatory, catatonic, etc. Acute psychosis has a low degree of nosological specificity. It may occur in the course of schizophrenia, affective disorders, organic disorders, pathological reactions in specific cultural contexts, or intoxications.

Chronic psychosis

The following negative symptoms are inherent to chronic psychosis: poor thinking and speech (alogia), abulia, flat affect, anhedonia, poor concentration, and social withdrawal. Positive symptoms are also frequently available, but lacking, however, the intensity and preoccupation of acute psychosis. A major exclusion to this is paraphrenia, a chronic psychosis without negative symptoms in which delusions predominate with steady and complex systematization and grandiose content, vigor, and vivid emotionality. Besides this rarer form, functioning in chronic psychosis is dependent mainly on the negative symptoms. Unlike the positive ones, with their morbid "creativity", negative symptoms result in the loss of normal functions. As a result, patients are secluded and have low motivation and energy, apathetic expressions, and poor hygiene. Their daily life is monotonous, and communication with others is reduced and formal (autisation), without any torment or boredom being caused by this. Cognitive decline, self-sufficiency, poverty, and dropping out of social networks, are all present. As contrasted to acute psychosis, which is an apparently pathological condition even according to the layperson, chronic patients appear to be idler and more neglected than ill. The syndrome occurs in the late phases of schizophrenia, but also in some other mental disorders with a chronic course, especially when combined with organic states and institutionalism.

Delirium

Delirium is an acute organic brain syndrome manifesting with: qualitative disturbances of consciousness with altered perceptions and orientation, regardless of levels of alertness (vigilance); misidentifications, illusions, and hallucinations, mostly visual ones; disturbed orientations towards time and space with well-preserved orientations towards the self; insomnia, or severe disturbances in the sleep-wake cycle; motor uneasiness, usually limited within the room; intense fear and, less frequently, ecstasy—or fluctuations between them; and marked autonomous signs. The delirious patient is commonly restless and fidgety. Their behavior is excited and helpless, combined with frightened looking around, staring, pointing, clinginess, pacing, or crumpling up the bed linens. Active attention and sleep are markedly disturbed. Diurnal fluctuations with exacerbated symptoms in the evening are characteristic. For alcohol delirium, flushing of the face, sweating, coarse tremor, and visual hallucinations—predominantly with visions of animals—as well as tactile hallucinations, and intense fear, are typical. The delirious patient is confused: misidentifying and being disoriented towards time and space, their self-orientation remains intact. The latter is disturbed in a more severe form of the syndrome, amentia. Establishing contact with a delirious patient is difficult, while in cases of amentia it is impossible.

Delirium is a sign of organic brain damage and may either arise out of severe physical diseases or intoxications, or follow general anesthesia. The syndrome is common in intensive care units, the most frequent kinds being alcohol delirium and delirium in vascular disease. After delirium, one's recollection of events is incomplete; and while recovery is possible, it is also quite common to find worsening of cognitive functions (dementia), or impairment of memory fixation and filling of memory gaps with confabulations (Korsakoff syndrome).

Dementia

Dementia is a chronic organic brain syndrome manifesting with: memory failure, predominantly for recent events—with relatively preserved, at least at the beginning, reproductions of events from the remote past; the impairment of intellect, and related thinking, judgment, calculation, orientation, learning, speech, and comprehension abilities; the loss of emotional control with frequent depressiveness, apathy, emotional instability, or euphoria with flat joking; and the decline of everyday habits, personal hygiene, and social behavior. If delirium is not superimposed, the patient's consciousness is not clouded. The main impairment is cognitive (predominantly in memory and intellect), but this is frequently masked by behavioral and emotional disturbances. The patient may look uneasy, scared, depressed, or neglected, and show signs of lability, flat joking, challenging others, or insolence. With their insight intact, usually in the early stages of dementia, patients may try to conceal their fading memory, or compensate for it with aids such as writing in a notebook. At later stages, however, difficulties with memory and judgment become apparent and may result in losing oneself, misidentifications, the distortion of memories, the impoverishment of thought content, habits deteriorating, and a need for constant supervision.

Many systemic and brain diseases may cause dementia. The main types in adults are Alzheimer's and vascular dementia. In Alzheimer's-type dementia, memory deficits are in the foreground, the course is gradual, and depression is frequent. In dementia with predominantly vascular etiology, the course is uneven, stepwise, with periods of worsening and improvement, marked diurnal dynamics, and emotional instability.

The main instrument in the recognition and assessment of psychopathology is the *interview*. Unlike in internal medicine, it is used not only for patient's history taking, but also for assessing the clinical condition, i.e., the interview and examination overlap with one another. The use of the interview as a therapeutic, not only assessing, instrument is unique to medicine. A session is an interview with the aim of therapeutic change through the interview situation itself. In the absence of external markers of validity for mental disorders ("psychiatric Wassermann")[198], the clinical interview remains the most reliable method for establishing phenomena in psychopathology, thus setting up the epistemological framework of psychiatry. The interview accounts for senses, meanings, and symbols; and for this reason, it is a second-order reality, as opposed to a first-order reality, accounting for the ontologically substantial qualities of things (e.g., the size or localization of a tumor). Through the interview, the (essential to psychiatric diagnosis) *meta-interpretation*, or, interpretation of the patient's interpretation of the world, is achieved. For the clinical assessment to reach its full value, however, what is shared by the patient needs to be balanced against data from other sources.

Among the necessary clinical skills and rules for conducting an interview,[69, 191] the most crucial one is probably keeping track of both content and process, e.g., the story and the way it is told. Keen attention to the process aspect of speech is one sign of a therapeutic attitude, requiring not only observation, but also self-observation. The clinician, trained in self-observation, is more prepared to view things sideways (from a *meta* position), maintain neutrality, and perceive the picture with its nuances, not from a black-and-white perspective. Standardized clinical assessments with structured interviews and scales contribute significantly to the reproducibility of descriptions, despite the epistemological limitations of positivist approaches to human experience, stemming from the fact that human beings, in the words of K. Schneider,[184] resist precise measurement. Besides, the applicability of structured instruments is debatable in many cultures of the Third World, where the talking context of the medical examination is unpopular.

4.2 Diagnosis and Case Formulation

Syndrome descriptions are integrated on higher levels into diagnoses and case formulation—hence, this phenomenology acquires categorization. Diagnosis is a central concept in psychiatry, practically defining the field. The diagnostic process of psychiatry has two aspects. One of them concerns recognizing symptoms and abnormal behaviors, considering their mutual relatedness, and referring to the diagnostic categories' criteria for classification. The other is associated with examining the patient holistically, finding the symptoms' corresponding links to personality, life path, and specific circumstances around illness, i.e., understanding the patient's individuality. This aspect is close to the real meaning of the word diagnosis, "to learn in depth" (from the Greek *diagignoskein*). The first approach assigns the patient to a larger group of people with similar pathologies (nomothetic approach), while the second one views them as a unique human subject (ideographic approach). While the first approach is mandatory in order to find regularities and provide care according to a definite standard, the latter is useful for understanding individual uniqueness in its own context and for developing a treatment plan. They refer to one another like Plato's ideal categories to the concreteness of Aristotle.

The principles of diagnostics rest on the concepts of *category* and *dimension*. The categorial approach adds a clinical state to an entity with clear boundaries, while the dimensional one refers it to a dimension where all individuals may be distributed on a continuum (axis) between two extremities. The gradual transition between norm and pathology is a rule, rather than an exclusion. Nature, according to Linnaeus[198], "does not make leaps". Clinical decisions, however, are usually categorial judgments requiring certain thresholds in the quantitative transition, which could discriminate disease cases from non-cases, with the inevitable loss of nuanced information at the expense of conceptual simplicity and facilitating clinical action. It is natural for patients to be distributed within certain dimensions—and for clinicians to think according to categories. Both approaches reflect the same phenomenon, but in different ways: either in its continuity, or as a separate entity.

The categorial approach differentiates pathology into groups with specific profiles, called disease units. The nosological unit, allegedly, links etiology, pathogenesis, clinical picture, course, and outcome. Such a monolithic and predictable entity is an extreme rarity in psychopathological diversity, and for this reason Jaspers[104] calls the ideal of a true nosology a Kantian idea, or a stimulus for scientific quest, however, not a reality. The grouping of diseases or cases is subject to either etiological (according to the causing agent), or syndromological (according to the clinical picture) principles. Purely etiological classifications are rare in medicine. With the relatively low-estimated specificity of syndrome pictures, in Kraepelin's time (during his dispute with Hoche), the notion of registers[35, 122] according to which the picture depends on the impaired level, not on an agent, originated. In disorientation, for instance, one's orientation to time is the first to be affected, followed by spatial orientation and, later on, by the orientation to oneself, with the disturbance's severity following the same course. This illustrates the hierarchy of the psyche's architecture, and its role in determining the diagnostic weight of impairments on its various levels. Diagnosing schizophrenia, for example, requires the exclusion of organic causes for symptoms.

The concepts of reliability and validity are related to the cognitive value of diagnostics and its instruments. Reliability refers to the reproducibility of the diagnosis, and reflects the degree of agreement by different clinicians in assessing the same clinical condition. Large international studies[100, 174, 221] find that reliability is higher for psychotic and affective symptoms, and lower for organic symptoms and personality traits, receding from the core to the periphery of the diagnostic entity. Validity reflects the degree to which diagnostic constructions can truly identify underlying pathologies. This remains an unsolved problem in psychiatry. Still, in 1843, Newmann notes that the recognition of disease is the recognition of its phenomenology, not of its essence.[198] In the absence of an approbated marker, the only certain way to achieve good knowledge about an ill person and correctly assign them to a group of people with a similar pathology is the clinico-descriptive approach. Symptoms are sometimes divided into basic (axial, primary) and reactive (secondary, compensatory) types, analogous to infections, where manifestations directly related to the agent may be concealed by unspecific symptoms of the reaction towards them.[25, 149] So, the choice of what constitutes an underlying pathology and what constitutes secondary or compensatory formation, is, in essence, a paradigmatic choice.

The *paradigms* are theoretical models containing not only scientific, but also ideological components.[149] There is broad consent that the test of a paradigm is its verification: if an attempt to refute it empirically fails, the paradigm is kept until a new verification can be performed; and if it does not stand the test, it is replaced by another one.[165] Thus, changing paradigms stimulate scientific development. Today's major paradigms in psychiatry are biological, psychodynamic, cognitive-behavioral, and bio-psycho-social—which allegedly balances out the reductionisms of the former three,[191] by somehow eclectically integrating factors from their domains into the conceptualization of psychopathology as a response to them.

Modern psychiatric diagnostics arose at the end of the 19th century. Until then, descriptions and labels of clinical pictures were exotic, based predominantly on symptom content. During the second half of that century, with the formidable development of the natural sciences and the accumulation of observations coming from large, asylum-type hospitals, Griesinger most clearly argued for the first time the differentiation of mental disorders as a separate class of diseases, unreducible only to brain pathology or degeneration.[35] Kraepelin's lasting merits are his dichotomy between dementia praecox (schizophrenia) and manic-depressive psychosis, his prioritization of illness course over syndrome presentation, and the clarity that he introduced into the clinical area. The term *endogenous* came into psychiatry when it was presented by Möbius as the initial definition of hereditary, later extending, however, to everything that cannot be traced back to known external causes. It is in opposition to *exogenic*, a term used by Bonhoeffer to denote toxic reactions and confused states due to physical causes, and, later, to *psychogenic* mental disorders, as well.[132] The division of pathology into these three major groups steadily marked the development of diagnostics throughout the 20th century.

The development of classifications was driven by the need to include cases that are beyond the clear boundaries of categorization, thus causing a peculiar *entropy* of psychiatric diagnoses. Borderline states, schizoaffective psychoses, cycloid psychoses, bouffée délirante, and the chronic hallucinatory psychosis of French authors,[48] are indicative of this process. Some classification schemes of the 20th century have played particular roles in clinical practice and in the development of psychiatric taxonomy. Jaspers[104] created the richest general psychopathology based on the phenomenological principle, offered clear criteria for exogenic and psychogenic disorders, and divided their clinical manifestations into processes, developments, and reactions. Based on a similar model, Schneider (Fig. 3) refined clinical thinking about schizophrenia, mood disorders, and personality disorders,[185] and described the first-rank symptoms of schizophrenia, making a huge impact on diagnostic criteria—although, with the relative superiority of positive symptoms over such manifestations as autism and thought disorganization, this probably served to distance diagnoses away from the presumed disease's validity. Additionally, Leonhard's typology[130] is particularly detailed and rich in clinical nuance, but has proven difficult to embrace for everyday use.

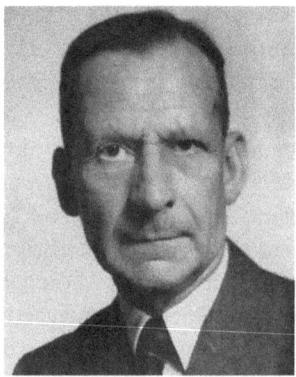

Fig. 3: Kurt Schneider (1887–1967) (Courtesy to Max-Planck-Institut für Psychiatrie, Historishes Archiv)

The classification of Snezhnevsky[189] is based on the combination of cross-sectional clinical pictures with the illness course, and on presumptions about predetermined changes in clinical states during different stages of the course. This school of thought was significantly influential in Eastern Europe for decades. Despite its clinical detailedness, it did not receive empirical support for its basic postulates (especially predetermination), and was discredited with its over-diagnosis of the schizophrenia spectrum, as well as its usage for repressive purposes in the former USSR.[64, 149, 190]

This development was witness to discord between traditions and schools of thought, although there is some evidence that this difference of opinion affected more nominal aspects of diagnostics, rather than its essence. In a 1908 retrospective assessment from 1908 with the contemporary diagnostic algorithm (CATEGO) of cases with dementia praecox and manic-depressive psychosis from the archive of the Munich psychiatric clinic where Kraepelin worked, Jablensky et al.[99] find that most of the states described in hospital records cover the criteria for the contemporary analogues of these diagnoses—schizophrenia and affective disorders.

Modern classifications, the ICD-10[222] and the DSM-5,[6] are the products of continuous research efforts at achieving international agreement[192], as demonstrated by the WHO studies on schizophrenia (Chapter 8). They do not represent nosologies, but are operational taxonomies subordinating diagnoses to a set of descriptive signs, rather than hypotheses of an underlying nature, predestined course, or outcome. Based on empirical data, they apply different principles to their different sections. In both classifications, the roles of quantitative criteria (i.e., symptom intensity, duration, or frequency), and the degree of subjective distress and dysfunction in different life areas, are decisive. In most sections, a cumulative (or polythetic) approach to recording symptoms is applied, and multiple diagnoses are admissible, with the exclusion of cases with some hierarchical domination, e.g., organic over other kinds of pathology.

The radical problem of these classifications is their as yet unproven validity. This causes uncertainty about the boundaries of the categories—we do not know whether phenomenological types correspond to underlying disturbances, or if such disturbances have no other range of manifestation (median phenotypes). There is sufficient evidence for a continuum between bipolar affective disorder and schizophrenia,[42] as well as between depression and anxiety—therefore, there is also a lack of grounds for their differentiation in its current form. An additional argument for this is the lack of specificity in treatments—they affect not diagnoses, but physiological or other dimensions. The polythetic approach is also problematic, with its requirement for a definite number of symptoms from a predefined checklist, leading to heterogeneity in the groups which exceed diagnostic thresholds[126] and artificial comorbidity. Other problem areas are the priority status of the nomothetical (label) alongside relative neglect of the ideographic (unique quality), as well as the prevalence of objectively observed behaviors over inner experiences. Consent regarding externally observed phenomena can be more easily achieved, and also leads to a heightened reliability of diagnosis; however, subjective experiences are closer to the essence of psychopathology.

For a more complex assessment, multiaxial approaches describing the patient's problems across different dimensions, and contextualizing pathology are suggested. A perspective variant of the World Psychiatric Association recommends the axes: I—clinical disorders (both mental and physical), II—disability, III—contextual factors, and IV—quality of life.[92, 93] Regardless of advancements in diagnostics, there are pronounced and multifaceted social and cultural limitations of its application. The ways in which psychiatric diagnoses are used are more indicative of socium than they are of psychiatric science and practices.[64] Yet, in spite of this, the consequences of *stigmatization* are universal across all cultures. Diagnosing, in itself, is a cognitive need which introduces clarity, albeit replacing understanding with a "pseudo-insight through terminology".[104] Diagnostics is also a manifestation of power,[178] although this is not always realized.

Case formulation is a personalized and flexible description with the aim of overcoming the limitations of diagnosis and achieving a thorough and contextualized insight into the ill person's condition. It is an additional method for making sense of, and integrating, psychopathology, by including unique peculiarities of the case, not just its assignment to a diagnostic category. Case formulation identifies significant problems and sifts out the secondary ones, discriminates between disease and illness behavior, offers deducibility and understanding of symptoms, and seeks consent for treatment. Ideographic formulation accounts for individual meanings of illness—putting them in the patient's own terms.[191] It is based on looking for *consent* between viewpoints (of the patient, his family, and the clinician) about the clinical state and its reasons. Such consent forms the core of case formulation, and is a precondition of therapeutic alliance. Unlike in medical diagnoses, with ideographic formulation pathology is not the only aspect being identified: the healthy resources of the patient are also found, including personal maturity, skills, sources of support, spiritual aspirations, and messages regarding expectations for recovery.[93]

An empirically simplified model of the transition from psychopathology to formulation can rest on what aspects of symptoms or treatment appear to be clinically unsatisfactory. The realistic first step in the process of formulation is the case's difficulty—because if a case can be inserted smoothly into a diagnostic category and its treatment goes efficiently, the clinician would rather not need a formulation. So, at the beginning, the question of why the case is not going well—and, the cause is commonly something that makes the case atypical or resistant—is asked. The next step is to clarify the reason for atypicality (e.g., quarrelsomeness in depression, erotomanic delusion, or overreaction to medications' side effects), which introduces an individual nuance to psychopathology. Like seemingly bizarre notions or casual slips of the tongue may be signs of covert conflict, so too in clinical practice can an inconvenient detail, evaded as being unnecessary, offer the key to understanding the case. The atypical (here, synonymous to individual) element of the picture frequently remains hidden, despite its conspicuousness, even from experienced clinicians.

What makes a case atypical usually coincides with what hinders recovery, i.e., sustains illness. Sustaining illness probably corresponds to certain needs, and makes one's illness safer than the responsibility of health. The reply to the question of why illness may be "preferable" becomes intelligible only by considering the atypical manifestation outside of its symptom assignment and placing it, instead, in the patient's context of daily and symbolic life. Only then may seemingly unexpected symptoms acquire meaning. This meaning is the basis for seeking out consent—not only for treatment, but also for what we find to be pathological and subject to change. Pre-formulation in psychopathology of this type is what makes for genuine, specifically individual, ideographic case formulation—and the subject matter of this formulation is closely tied to culture.

5 The Culture-Psychopathology Relationship

> What we observe is not nature itself, but nature exposed to our method of questioning.
>
> *W. Heisenberg*

Culture and psychopathology share common characteristics. They have a common ontology: both are over-biological systems and ways of interpreting either collective (culture) or individual (psychopathology) experience and behavior. They also have a common epistemology: their leading traits are not entirely realized consciously by participants, and may be more apparent to an external observer, while insight into both of them requires putting oneself in "other people's shoes". Culture, undoubtedly, influences all aspects of symptomatology: from its genesis, manifestation, and recognition, to the meaning attributed to it, and the way help is sought out. Many cultural distinctions have biological reasons. Sickle cell anemia is most prevalent in the Mediterranean and Africa, and though it protects against malaria, it unfortunately predisposes patients to psychosis. Tularemia is also quite frequently found in the Mediterranean, and it plays a role in the rise of some psychoses, as well. Annual hours of sunshine have a direct effect on depression and suicides and are at the basis of vast differences between populations at the equator, moderate latitudes, and the poles. Infectious diseases historically have played a considerable role in the rise of different psychopathological forms, as well as in their alteration in pace with changes or the eradication of diseases. The massive prevalence of infectious diseases in the Third World, and absence in developed countries, sustains even today great dissimilarities in these two worlds' pathologies. The difference between catatonias (Chapter 8) is just one such example.

The history of interweaving between culture and psychopathology is inseparable from the history of views about mental illness and caring for the mentally ill. Since ancient times, at the folk level of all cultures, there have been intuitive ways for explaining psychological deviations according to respective cosmogonies. Regardless of scientific progress, the pre-historical lack of distinction between medicine, magic, and religion regarding attitudes about the mentally ill, is, in a sense, still preserved in the present day.

5.1 Historical Steps of Interweaving

As early as in the third millennium BCE, sleep therapy, music therapy, amulet wearing, dancing, and drawing were applied in the temple of Imhotep the healer in Memphis. Around 2000 BCE, in Mesopotamia, according to the Code of Hammurabi, priest-healers dealt with diseases of the mind that were attributed to demons, while "lay" healers dealt with far less prestigious physical injuries. This is the earliest known division between mental and physical symptoms.[166] Records on Egyptian papyrus from 1550 BCE mention depression. In Biblical texts, there are trustworthy descriptions of the severe depression of King Saul, Nebuchadnezzar's psychotic fear of turning into a wolf (lycanthropy), Ezekiel's coprophagy, and David's simulation. The reaction to David's successful simulation is indicative of the scope of mental illness in ancient times: "Achish said to his servants: 'Look at that man! He is insane! Why bring him to me? Am I so short of madmen that you have to bring this fellow to carry on like this in front of me?'" (First Book of Samuel 21: 14–15). In general, mental deviations were then accepted as the product of physical causes or supernatural forces. This division, under different forms, continued for centuries. According to the Talmud, with its particular wealth of psychological interpretations, madness is a punishment for sins which may be alleviated by sharing, while dreams release one's suppressed desires.

In Ancient Greece, according to Homer, the ancient healer Melampus would prescribe yarrow for overtly psychotic states, something to be ironized later on in Greek comedies. Herodotus, describing the atrocities of a Persian king, writes that "...the spirit may not be healthy if the body is ill".[220] In the temples of Asclepius, usually close to thermal springs, sleep therapy was applied in surroundings full of luxury and suggestibility, similarly to the modern spa industry. Hippocrates (4th century BCE) considered physiological anomalies to be the basis for mental disorders. He reliably described depression, and classified personalities according to the four somatic liquids. Plato describes the soul as a rider of two horses—one noble, and the other one driven by primary passions, with the rider balancing between them.[74] And, according to Aristotle, most of the creative personalities are melancholic, while the plays of Aristophanes demonstrate free associations. Along with the scope of the epoch's ideas, practical activities were also carried out[215], with an emphasis on private practice, particularly in Athens. Simultaneously, the severely mentally ill were tied up and isolated, a practice that did not spare even the king of Sparta.[35] Soranus of Ephesus in the 2nd century CE insisted on a humane attitude towards patients, applied predominantly through psychological treatment, and furthermore recommended

Tab. 2: Axes for assessing a mentally ill person in the Roman tribunal, 1st century BCE

Dimension	Content
Nomen	clan/tribe, region, ties
Natura	sex, race, marital status, age, physique
Victus	education, habits/lifestyle
Fortuna	rich/poor, free/slave, social class
Habitus	appearance
Affectio	passions, emotions, temperament
Studium	interests
Consilium	motivation
Factum	job history
Casus	significant life events
Orationes	form and content of speech

the alkyl waters of the town for mania—18 centuries later, high concentrations of lithium were discovered there.

In Rome, physical methods of treatment like baths, massage, music, and sometimes light electroshock from eels, were applied. In the Roman tribunals, a scheme attributed to Cicero for assessing the mentally ill on 11 axes—an example of a multiaxial assessment in cultural context—was introduced (Tab. 2). It was used throughout the Roman Empire and, centuries later, in some Celtic monasteries. Within Roman jurisprudence, the category of insanity was introduced, along with its reasons—furor, mentecaptio, melancholia—which, in the Justinian Code, also included insania, dementia, moria, mentecaptio, fatuitas, and affect.[183]

Aretaeus of Cappadocia (1st–2nd centuries CE), an eclectic medical philosopher, was the first to describe manic-depressive illness, emphasizing that not everyone with a mental disorder also displayed imbecility—a fact left without sufficient clarity even until the 20th century.[166] He also demonstrated rare concern for the state of ill persons, in contrast to the torture that they were frequently subjected to. Hunger and whipping are recommended by Cornelius Celsus (1st century CE), "because such is the fate of the lunatic" (*quoniam is dolus insanientis est*)[35]—a long-sustained and, apparently, culturally acceptable argument for torturing and, later on, burning alive mentally ill people.

In the 7th century, the first known psychiatric ward was opened in Baghdad. During the age of the caliphates, especially under the Abbasid dynasty, attitudes among Arabs about the mentally ill was more humane than in Western Europe at the same time.[151] The works of Galen and Aristotle were translated and studied, and the Arabic translation of Hippocrates by Constantine the African in Salerno in particular gave new impetus to the idea that the brain is the primary cause of mental diseases.[14] Avicenna (11th century) would relate inner experiences to physiology and develop a system for recording emotional changes through the pulse rate.

From the beginning of the 14th century, hospitals and asylums for the mentally ill began opening up in Western and Northern Europe, firstly in Valencia, Spain, and shortly afterwards in Uppsala, Sweden, and Elbing, Germany. In London, mentally ill people were kept as early as the 13th century at Bedlam, an abbey later transformed into a hospital that would become emblematic for the field of psychiatry. These asylums originated as shelters for wandering mentally ill persons who had, commonly, been expelled along with the plague-stricken and lepers by city authorities. In Frankfurt am Main, for example, the mentally ill were loaded onto boats and rafts, and pushed down river out of the city walls.[35] In Germany and other northern countries, asylums were called houses for the mad (Tall Houses). In many such places in Switzerland, Spain, and France, wine was regularly given to the residents. During the Middle Ages, despite later evaluations, the care given to the mentally ill of Western Europe was better than in subsequent centuries. The themes of compassion and spiritual healing penetrated steadily into the intellectual climate of the era, particularly through its poetry. Care for patients in the early years of London's Bedlam was so valuable that, not infrequently, vagrants would snatch away the plates from the hands of the mentally ill so that they could make use of the privileges of a hospital stay instead.

Advancements in the natural sciences during the Renaissance stimulated the development of ideas about the connection between the brain and mental pathology. Around the 14th century, at the dawn of the Renaissance, the persecution and burning of "witches" at stakes began, leading to the largest-scale extermination of mentally ill people in history[35, 58, 166] (along with mentally healthy persons, once confessions had been extorted from them). At that time, a severe plague killed around half of the population in Europe, and the mass conviction that it was a punishment for sins was imposed. The ideology of the witch hunt was shaped at the end of the 14th century by Innocent VIII's papal bull and the grotesque writing of two Dominican monks, *Malleus Maleficarum* (The Hammer of Witches), published in 1487, which became a manifesto for the persecutions. It endorsed the dogma that mental disease is caused by seduction and seizure by the devil, while torture and burning were accepted as the means for driving the devil away from the body, thus ensuring the immortality of the soul.[166] More humane methods such as expelling demons (exorcism) and sheltering in monasteries were also applied. In the 16th and 17th centuries, in contrast to demonology, and in parallel with ideological steps such as mechanistic (Descartes and Bacon) and deterministic (Hobbes and Locke) teachings, as well as closely following the introduction of empiricism to science (Newton), notions about mental disorders as *medical diseases* gained prevalence.[35]

Treatment methods included diets, vomiting, warm baths, bloodletting, applying leeches or warm animal organs, e.g., a lamb's lung to the shaved head of a patient, expensive amulets, rituals, and herbs. Probably the most widely used psychopharmacological agent before contemporary psychopharmacology (besides alcohol), was the hellebore plant, taken as an infusion for centuries, independently, in different European countries.[35] In Eastern Europe, the care for mentally ill people was predominantly assumed by monasteries. During the Ottoman Empire's period of flourishing under Suleiman the Magnificent, in Istanbul a very well laid out and luxurious medical facility for the mentally ill was opened in 1560. At that time, a typical scene in the asylums of Western Europe featured dark premises with chains and dirty residents, frequently smeared with feces, being treated with immersions in water, rotations on chairs, wheels, or beds, strait jackets, emetics, etc. In Bedlam, there were days for paid visits, when the audience would watch patients in cages for entertainment.

The Enlightenment left a profound imprint on attitudes towards mental illness by removing the chains of the mentally ill—in Paris, Pinel and his former patient Pussin, who would later become superintendent, did this in Bicêtre in 1794 and in La Salpêtrière in 1795. This event, groundbreaking in psychiatry, was followed by further developments, marked by rationalism and the humanistic ideas of the epoch.[58] Liberating patients allowed for the observation of their natural conditions, leading to the richness of 19th-century clinical descriptions. Therapeutic communities were established, having been pioneered by the York Retreat of W. Tuke, a Quaker and tea merchant who laid down a strict regime, reproducing protestant values and the atmosphere of an average bourgeois family: rigid order, hygiene, daily chores, self-help, and a ban on violence. Here the foundations of so-called moral therapy, characterized by sanctions and encouragements which resonated with the puritanical views of the age, were laid. The Marquis de Sade fell victim to this approach when he was hospitalized by Esquirol for immoral behavior. The term psychiatry came into life in 1808, although it had already arisen as a medical discipline as early as the 17th century; still, it came not from abstract theories, but as a response to the practical necessity of introducing order in the asylums. The first legal regulations for involuntary detainment in asylum, developed in France and England,[154] established social engagement and control over psychopathology, converting it into a cultural metaphor of the link between civilization and madness.[58]

During the first half of the 19th century, in England social discontent over inhumane conditions in the asylums spread, resulting in the establishment of a system for non-restraint. In Germany at that time, abstract (in theory) Naturphilosophie was combined with "pedagogical" approaches in practice, including disciplining, use of the straight chair, sacks, wheels, cages, and masks preventing grimacing, immersion in cold water, and routine vomiting and bloodletting. The debate between the psychic and somatic schools of thought, characteristic for the time, reflected the dualism between mechanistic theories and romanticism in philosophy and the predominant views on life. In all of Europe during the 19th century, new mental hospitals were opened and positivistic observation was stimulated. Besides the mentally ill, these hospitals also sheltered patients with severe neurological diseases, particularly dementia, epilepsy, and general paresis of the insane, as well as criminals and deviants. By attributing many antisocial and immoral behaviors to mental diseases, 19th-century psychiatry was transformed into a victim of its own nosology and propaganda, helping magistrates to send criminals into asylums rather than putting them on trial.[166]

The asylum-type of hospitals appeared to be desirable places, as they offered food and shelter, and the number of their residents was constantly rising due to poverty and unemployment, among other reasons. The general principle of care was simple, good-minded paternalism. At the same time, hospitals in Russia (Tall Houses) were considered to be worse than prisons or labor camps.[35] Disappointment with moral therapy gave rise to new theories about heredity, degeneration, and brain pathology. These theories were in line with the atmosphere of the time: degeneration followed Prussia's victory in 1870, the Paris Commune, and the bourgeoisie fear of the impoverished and degenerate masses, while the domestic endorsement of neurasthenia in the USA was in unison with overt tenseness about the competitive nature of business. In Bulgaria (and some other Eastern Orthodox countries), the term *soul disease* (with 'soul' in place of 'mental')[117] can be traced back to medieval texts in Old Church Slavonic, where it denotes not only madness, but also ignorance and brutalization.[193] Such stigmatization of mental illness as a disease of the soul, and its equation with intellectual or moral ailments, is intrinsic to Orthodox culture—and was later held up in the parlance of Bulgarian psychiatry with the paradoxically anti-stigmatizing argument that the prefix *psycho* was absent.[154]

The nosological approach from the fifth edition of Kraepelin's textbook (1896) and Freud's psychoanalysis arose almost simultaneously at the end of the century, and exerted a decisive, *parallel* influence on psychiatry and culture throughout

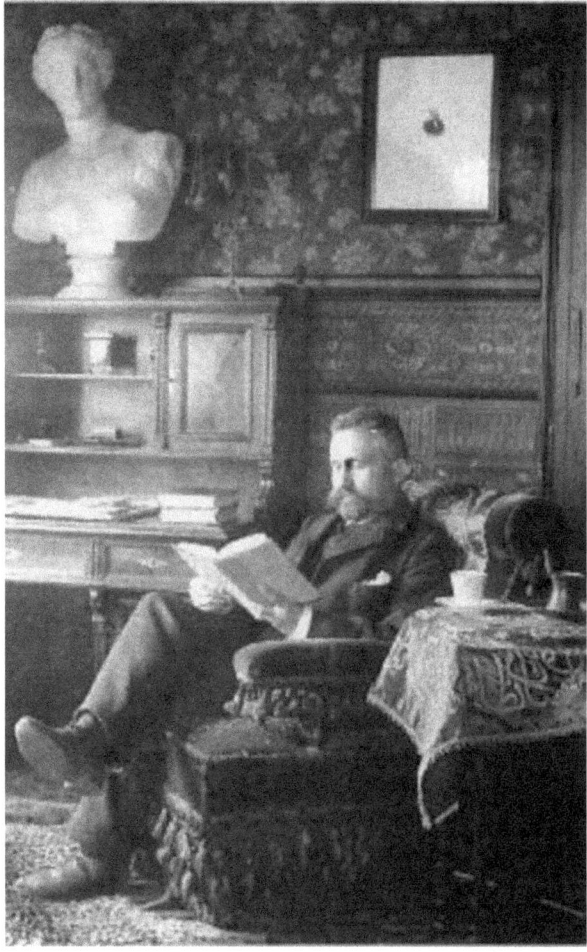

Fig. 4: Emil Kraepelin (1856–1926), around the time of his voyage to Java, 1903 (Courtesy to Max-Planck-Institute für Psychiatrie, Historisches Archiv)

the 20th century (Fig. 4, Fig 5). Mental illness behavior has always absorbed cultural fashions and models. Like hysteria in the 19th century was enigmatic of the artistic *fin de siècle*, so in the 20th century were anxiety neurosis, hypochondria, and borderline states allegorical to shaken identity, existential insecurity, and inner emptiness. Being *nervous* or *depressed* became social idioms, explanations, alibis, and metaphors, or wielded privilege. The young "rebel without a cause"

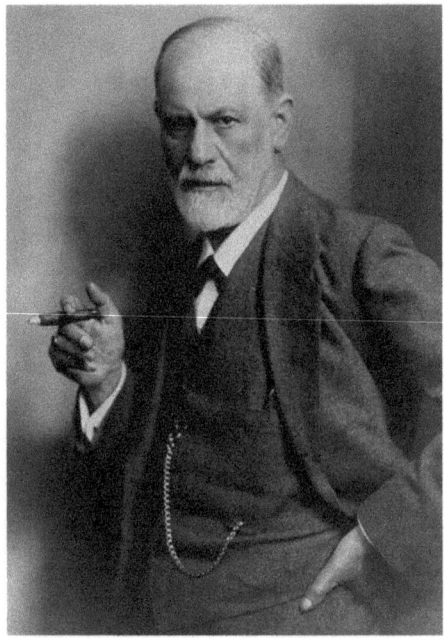

Fig. 5: Sigmund Freud (1856–1939) (Courtesy to Getty Images)

of the 1950s and 60s was a version of the melancholic Romantic poet. Having a *chick shrink* in the 20th century was as fashionable as staying in a tuberculosis sanatorium in the Alps a hundred years earlier. And, after Bismarck's development of the then-best insurance system in the world, the illness model called "disability neurosis" by German psychiatrists was formed.[183]

In the 20th century, the culture–psychopathology relationship acquired a dual directedness: not only was psychopathology determined to have its own cultural interpretations, but culture also obtained psychopathological interpretations. Thus, psychoanalysis associates early Christianity with ambivalence and rebellion against the father; capitalism with an anal character, individualization, and an obsession with hard work beyond what is needed for living (unintelligible from the viewpoint of many communities); communism is soaked in irrationality, inferiority complexes, and double-faced attitudes to the bourgeoisie ("with a bottle of Martell in one hand, and the writings of Lenin in the other");[94] democracy offers individual freedom and development, but also loneliness; and authoritarianism is instilled by neurotic sadomasochistic needs, the need for dependence and an escape from freedom.[63] Psychoanalysis changed the intellectual climate of the 20th century, while progress made in clinical psychiatry and neuroscience supported changing attitudes about the mentally ill. Technological advances provided new treatments, such as malariotherapy, psychosurgery, insulin coma therapy, electro-convulsive therapy, and psychopharmacology, and parallel developments in psychodynamic and cognitive-behavioral therapy were also achieved.

Commonly throughout history, not all scientific achievements have had their unequivocal applications in practice. At the beginning of the 20th century in the USA and in the 1930s in Sweden and Germany, mass sterilizations of the mentally ill were carried out with the arguments of disease heredity and eugenics. Besides this, from 1939 to 1945 in Germany some 220,000 to 269,000 mentally ill people, half of them schizophrenic (accounting for between 73 and 100 % of all patients with schizophrenia in Germany at the time), including children, were murdered via gas chamber (carbon monoxide) or injection (e.g., scopolamine)—all of them were killed after receiving psychiatric assessments of their eligibility.[205] This program, called T-4, was promoted by Rüdin and other psychiatric experts with the belief that schizophrenia is a simple Mendelian inherited disease. It was, ironically, initially supported by the Rockefeller Foundation.

Greater efficiency of treatments altered the scope of mental health services in the second half of the 20th century and facilitated the process of deinstitutionalization and psycho-social rehabilitation. As a cultural product of the powerful movement for human rights and changing societal attitudes to mental illness, starting in the 1960s antipsychiatry advocates claimed that mental illness was a myth, while the aim of psychiatry was to encourage social control through the identification and sanctioning of deviants.[203] Among the milder antipsychiatric analogues today are the libertarian movements that combine ecological, Marxist, and psychoanalytical views. Civilization, according to Foucaut,[58] represses not only human instincts but also all forms of transcendence, and psychiatry serves this repression by coercing the mentally ill to interiorize bans and control, thus allegorically taking the physical bars from the psychiatric hospital windows and moving them into their individual world. The relevance of topics such as stigma, discrimination, the need for cultural sensitivity in the treatment of people from other cultures, and recovery from severe mental illness as a leading paradigm of psycho-social rehabilitation ever increases. Rehabilitation alters the pattern of psychiatric care, and its essence is nothing less than the literal integration of psychopathology into the patient's cultural environment.

5.2 Symptom Formation

Interest towards manifestations of psychopathology present in other cultures can be traced back to the colonial era, and is associated with an anthropological curiosity about the savage, a boom in the natural sciences, and the influence of Darwinism. This process transformed from anthropological descriptions into a focus on what is culture specific or exotic from a Eurocentric viewpoint, and then to the ethnographic approach with its emphasis on meanings and context. In 1903, Kraepelin traveled to Java, Indonesia, where he observed patients in the large colonial hospital asylum on the island. His general conclusion was that, despite civilizational distinctions, the severe pathologies he witnessed were clinically similar to what could have been observed in German hospitals at the time.[107] This voyage is considered the onset of transcultural psychiatry, also called comparative (a term, preferred by Kraepelin himself), cross-cultural, or ethno-psychiatry.[145]

The aim of the discipline, regardless of its designation, is the identification and explanation of relationships which exist between mental disorders and these psycho-social characteristics that differentiate across nations, ethnicities, or cultures. There is relative agreement that the influence of these characteristics is greater on reactive and neurotic states than it is on major "endogenous" diseases.[146] Nevertheless, the largest-scale studies on the influence of sociocultural factors on mental illness were conducted precisely about schizophrenia (Chapter 8). The development of transcultural psychiatry gained momentum during the 60s with descriptions of culture specific states, unusual to Europe and North America, and continued through the WHO collaborative studies in the 70s and the 80s on schizophrenia, with the notable contribution of Jablensky.[100, 101] The field has since acquired new dimensions, including elaborative efforts to make use of culturally sensitive classifications and cultural axes in the assessment of psychopathology and its ethnographic focus on the context of local meanings and metaphors.[203, 204]

The main, yet unresolved, debate in transcultural psychiatry is currently one between biological universalism and cultural relativism.[106] According to the *universalist* approach, the biological core of psychopathology is universal, and the role of culture is only pathoplastic, while according to the anthropologically *relativist* approach, culture is more deeply involved in the etiology and forms of illness expression. The study of universal phenomena presumes being able to describe them with structured instruments and from the viewpoint of an external observer (*etic* approach); on the other hand, idiopathic phenomena can be freely observed and described from the viewpoint of a certain group's

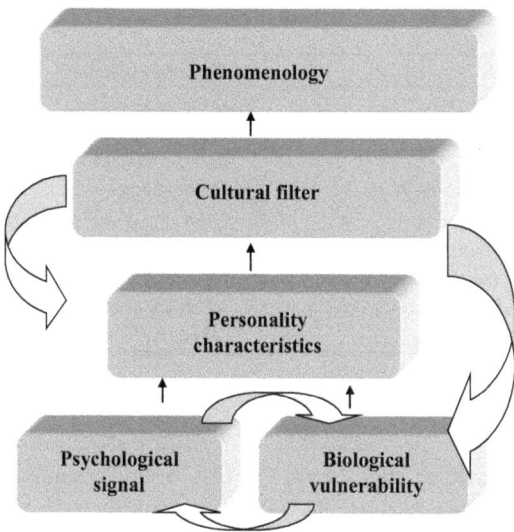

Fig. 6: Symptom formation in psychopathology

participant (*emic* approach). These terms come from phonetics and indicate universal or specific phonemes. The universalist approach is considered adequate regarding data about severe mental disorders,[100] while the relativist one is more applicable to culture specific syndromes and a number of dissociative states.

Culture and psychopathology interact with each other even at the level of symptom formation, in which culture acts as a *filter* for morbid signals (Fig. 6). When biological, these signals have no subjective meaning and are semantically undetermined ("primordial soup").[20] Their configuration according to cultural codes is realized through both individual peculiarities and the cultural milieu, which, for their part, may have an inverse effect on signals, displaying some selectivity. Molecules and amino acids do not carry cultural messages; it is only through their processing of the personality and cultural layers of symptom formation that they can cause phenomena with semantic meaning. This kind of meaning is apparent on two levels: in the individual recognition and interpretation of senses and experiences and in the expression of this interpretation in front of others, including the clinician.[20, 168] For this reason, psychopathology is meta-interpretation (Chapter 4): the clinical interpretation of patients' individual interpretations of lived experiences. This epistemological perusal should not omit the specification that descriptive categories—from ancient metaphysical

Tab. 3: Basic differences in psychopathology between cultures

Traditional cultures	Modern cultures
Paternalism	Informed consent
Obligation to live	Right to die
Collective anxiety	Individual distress
Somatizations and dissociations	Depressions
Uncommon suicides	High suicide rate
Low rate of alcohol, high rate of cannabis use	High rate of addictions
More favorable course of schizophrenia	More unfavorable course of schizophrenia
Infectious diseases, organic states, catatonias	Obsessive-compulsive disorder, anorexia

denominations to the operational criteria of current classifications—are rooted in language and culture and, because of this, are also loaded with symbolic meanings which have nothing to do with brain signals.

Psychopathology may also find its cause in psychological signals, as they transform into symptoms—like any human experience—through physiological participation. Like biological signals, psychological ones are not directly realized as psychopathological phenomena, but are rather twisted and edited by personality peculiarities and culture. Unlike biological signals however, they are loaded with semantic meaning from their first incidence (e.g., trauma) and are not subject to radical remaking. Depending on the nature of the signal, its semantic expression may be less influenced by the layers of personality and culture, or may even bypass them, and more directly access its phenomenology and interpretations. Thus, in bypassing the inner cultural filter, the symptom's semantic meaning is directly inserted within a wider cultural interpretative space.

Some idiopathic expressions of illness[142] are unintelligible outside of the context of local meanings and local *idioms* for experiencing distress—metaphors, behavioral models, or physical symptoms. These models suggest that syndromes are constructed out of cultural experience and do not draw only from an assumed universal underlying core. Social constructioning requires an awareness of the cultural matrix in which the syndrome arises because psychopathology's manifestations are idiomatic and do not follow known syndromic patterns. Beyond the constructivist model, culture's influence on psychopathology has many faces (Tab. 3). In many cultures in the Third World, for instance, depression manifests more frequently with somatization masks and the experience of shame instead of guilt (Chapter 9), while obsessive-compulsive disorder is rare and anorexia is almost unheard of (Chapter 10), yet catatonias are more frequent and the course of schizophrenia is more favorable (Chapter 8). At the same time, dissociative states and magical explanations are commonplace there (Chapter 7) and may attach a quasi-psychotic pattern to nonpsychotic conditions.[153] Bioethical concepts such as informed consent and patient autonomy fall entirely within the framework of cultural relativism,[151] particularly when attempts are made to apply them in communities where decisions are made not by the individual, but by the clan, and marriages are usually prearranged by parents.

These differences illustrate the problems associated with cross-cultural diagnostics, and the need for clinicians to possess cultural sensitivity.[145] From another standpoint, modern psychiatric diagnostics has its intellectual basis in mechanistic philosophy, the notion that illness is an ontological reality, and the role played by the central nervous system in psychopathology.[142] These impose an objective approach and descriptive language about the phenomena liberated from any moral, personal, or situational nuances. In this way, neutrality and verification are achieved, however, at the expense of losing the phenomena's contextuality and sense of cultural meaning.

Cultural specifics in the manifestation of symptoms are due to the influence of culture on psychological processes (Chapter 2). Many aspects of human psychology are universal because the need for coping with biological imperatives is universal.[173] Among these are cultural stereotypes and group prejudices. Biological differences, e.g., in enzymes or related to skull size, can directly reflect onto cultural differences. An example of this kind of interaction between biological and cultural factors is antisocial personality disorder in boys with low levels of the monoamine oxidase inhibitor (MAOI) and traumatic childhoods, as compared to the absence of antisocial pathologies with low levels of MAOI—however, this only applies in cases also lacking traumatic experiences during childhood.[181] Culture leaves its imprint on temperament, social cognition, language (not just as a means for expression, but as the way we think and feel, according to the Sapir-Whorf hypothesis),[219] locus of control, individual and collective identity, and, thence, on symptoms manifesting through these psychological processes. The determination of abnormality itself is culturally colored. Culture has become a central concept in psychiatric theory and practice.[82]

A basic problem we now face is how to incorporate it into psychopathological formulation. At the same time, though, clinical cultural sensitivity may prove to be misleading. Attributing cultural labels (e.g., Maori or Muslims) also places political and identity markers and may cloud, instead of outline, the individual characteristics that are decisive in psychopathology.[169] Misunderstandings about abnormal behavior in the relevant cultural context may lead to over-diagnoses, under-diagnoses, or erroneous diagnoses, with all their respective consequences.

6 Mysticism and Psychopathology

> God has no religion.
>
> *M. Gandhi*

Religions, superstitions, and mystical knowledge have accompanied mankind since prehistory, when we acquired the unique ability to recognize our own experiences. Their appearance was probably connected to that of an awareness about mortality (Chapter 2). They are not simply an irrevocable part of culture, but something which arose simultaneously alongside it, shaping it too. Beliefs in the afterlife and miracles satisfy the primary human needs for explanation, meaning, and consolation—these are just as archaic as the biological imperatives of sex, hunger, thirst, survival, or acceptance.

In physical and mental illness, the role of religion and paranormality increases due to the limitations of the biomedical model's neglecting the experiential aspect of illness.[74, 84] Descartes called the human body a machine, and this attribute continues to influence the development of medicine even today.[204] Following this logic is the notion that organs, like the components of a machine, can be repaired—with physicians acting as mechanics and technicians. Contemporary technological medicine does not differentiate the subjective illness experience from the objective picture, and, as it is preoccupied more with measurements than meaning, it doesn't take patients' beliefs very much into account either.[84] The main reason behind the steadiness of magical beliefs during illness is that they add meaning to the experience of being ill. From the viewpoint of scientific medicine, this meaning is irrelevant, but for some people would be more acceptable than a casual genetic mutation or metabolic fault.

Although the basic functions of religions and paranormal beliefs appear to be similar, they differ in essential ways, including their relatedness to psychopathology and illness behavior. Major, normative *religions* are shared by large masses of people, increase the adaptability of individuals and the community,[74] and have their own moral codes. *Paranormal beliefs* are shared by small groups, usually within closed subcultures, and cause, as a rule, the isolation of people from the rest of society, as well as serving utilitarian aims. Religion responds to the need for meaning and consolation, while the paranormal does this for the need to master primary anxiety and reach a certain outcome through a miracle.

6.1 Religion and Psychopathology

Religiosity creates religions, not vice versa.[161] The religious feeling is a basic need that originates in survival and reproductive instincts. The supernatural is not an ontological datum, but a creation of the human need for it, or, as E.A. Poe puts it, all religions arise from "lies, fear, greediness, imagination, and poetry". A belief in the afterlife is the core of every religion. The afterlife is a sui generis continuation of life, which is why genuine religiosity is the endorsement, not denial, of life. The sense and strength of the major religions are rooted in the ontological continuum between life, death, and their extensions. This continuum is internally inherent to man, whose name (*human*) originates from the Latin word for earth (*humus*), symbolizing the beginning and the end. Religiosity helps to overstep the bounds of reason and overcome hesitation via confidence in a supra-individual stance ("above-personal will"[161]), although its moral limitations also serve as a neurotic factor. The idea of God is regarded by A. Toynbee[207] as the highest spiritual achievement in human history and major driving force behind it—which attaches, according to M. Eliade,[52] a trans-historical meaning to the otherwise meaningless tragic events in history. The *spiritual* dimension overlaps with religiosity, especially in the major monotheistic religions, without, however, coinciding with it. Religion has specific behavioral, denominational, and doctrinal characteristics that are associated with faith in a supernatural power, while spirituality is entirely oriented towards the meaning of life and its connection with transcendence—which may or may not be related to religion.

The content of faith is not an indicator of a believer's health or pathology. The discrepancy between the impossibility of verifying such content and certain claims about pathology is reflected in the notion that normal religious beliefs refer to things that are not subject to objective examination, and therefore do not contradict everyday experience. On the contrary, with pathological beliefs, the opposite is frequently the case.[161] In clinical practice or research, the question of whether God exists is irrelevant; what is relevant concerns the role of faith in illness and treatment. Psychiatry has maintained a traditionally ambivalent attitude towards religion and has also been inclined to pathologize religiosity and spirituality; the field has only recently recognized the empirically positive influence of religiosity on illness.

Religiosity offers consolation and connection (*re-ligare*—connect again) as an antidote to existential dread and a spiritual vacuum; having a deep collective sense of community survival ("the social character of religious feeling"[161]) improves both adaptiveness and individual integrity.[74, 161] The religious personality is clearly differentiated from God, while the experience of fusion with Him, common in the ecstatic states of various cults, is regarded as pathological by the believers themselves. The healing role of religion is acknowledged in different ways. Freud defines religion as a universal neurosis and sign of personal immaturity, but at the same time underlines its protective function against neuroticism on an individual level.[62] Jung associates it with defense mechanisms.[109] Due to its protective function, religious conversion during psychosis is sometimes interpreted as a compensatory formation, introducing equilibrium to the inner world which has been disturbed by the psychosis.[135] Studies show that religiosity among psychiatric patients in closed wards resembles in prevalence that of the general population from which these patients originate.[122, 125] In meta-analysis, religiosity correlates with positive mental health,[103] and is also a protective factor against depression in old age. Religiosity leads to faster improvement in cases of severe depression,[120] and is associated with better ambulatory status and lower depressiveness in elderly people recovering from surgical interventions.[167] True religiosity additionally prevents against suicide and alcohol or drug addiction.

At the same time, religiosity and mental illness interplay in different ways: religion may precipitate, resemble (in ecstasy or other mystical states), complicate, or provide shelter from illness. In the ancient texts of Abrahamic religions sharing a common root—Judaism, Christianity, and Islam—madness is often described naturalistically, but the privilege of having a direct relationship with God is also pointed out not too infrequently. The Bible offers different instances of psychopathological manifestations in the Old Testament, such as psychotic depression in Saul, treated with David's playing on the lyre, or Nebuchadnezzar's regressive psychosis and simulation of mental illness by David ("So he pretended to be insane, scratching on doors and drooling down his beard", First Book of Samuel 21: 13). These are only in addition to numerous other mentions of miraculous cures performed by Jesus in the New Testament (altogether 41 of them appear in the four Gospels) through expelling spirits or simply using words and touch, while the Pharisees insinuated His possession by a demon (John). The topical themes found in the eternal books of sin, guilt, redemption, power, obedience, fidelity, treachery, lust, or homosexuality (Leviticus) are steadily inserted into the content of illness experiences. An excessive preoccupation with sin and guilt is characteristic for patients with depression, while excessive conscientiousness is present in patients with obsessive-compulsive disorder or dysthymia—its total absence characterizes antisocial personalities. Existential issues may assume a ruminative and philosophizing pattern, e.g., "Why is the pious Job so mercilessly punished by God, if He is really just?"

Throughout the Old Testament, and in other monotheistic traditions, illness is justified as punishment for one's sins. Paul the Apostle reformulates this

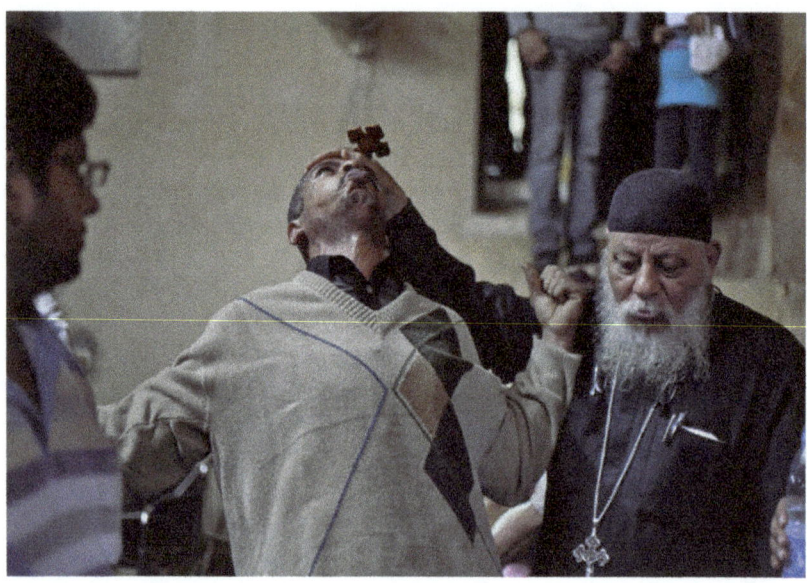

Fig. 7: An Arab Orthodox Coptic priest exorcises a Muslim compatriot

conception as a privileged display of God's mercy towards ailing and ill people, thus initiating the Christian tradition to eulogize suffering. Prayers were used intensively as treatment until the 4th century, but this practice later declined.[103, 104] Religious moralistic analogies for health and illness are similar to those developed by the school of psychics from the 19th century, yet Griesinger warned against religious and sectarian tendencies in psychologizing pathology.[121] Religious healing cults have flourished across centuries and until the present day, with their leaders typically being charismatic antisocial personalities, mentally ill (most frequently, paraphrenic), charlatans, or some combination of the three. Religious healing (Fig. 7) may indeed bring about the temporal alleviation of some mental or physical suffering, but it could also cause the loss of autonomy and falling into states similar to psychosis.

Mystical *ecstasy* is an extreme form of religious experience marked by an inexpressible sense of being able to discern beyond the obvious meanings of things, achieving oneness with God or another transcendent power, widening of the consciousness, and accessing non-conventional awareness like insight or creative wisdom;[103] and it is commonly accompanied by enthralling eroticism. These signs may also be incidental in acute psychosis with cycloid pattern, especially if coinciding with sudden and intense delusional mood. On the phenomenological level, psychosis and mystical states are difficult to differentiate. Although formal thought disorder and auditory hallucinations are more characteristic of psychosis, and visual hallucinations—of mystical experiences, other discriminating factors are more relevant. Mystical ecstasy, usually found in extremely religious, immature people who are also prone to dissociations, is in harmony with the cult context—it cannot be separated from it, nor does it cause any recognized dysfunction. Conversely, psychosis completely rules such behavior out of the context of religious experience and does disturb functioning. Ecstatic states are sometimes, allegedly, associated with revelations (the Prophet Muhammad, Saint Ignatius) or creative achievements (Dostoevsky), and are consciously sought by some, e.g., dervishes and Sufis, through combinations of rituals and sometimes with the help of psychoactive substances. In his *Canon of Medicine*, Avicenna describes the role of music and self-absorption in achieving religious ecstasy, in the same manner later practiced by vocalist sects: the follower of the cult is seated on the ground, repeating the name of Allah until all movements of the tongue and lips cease, and the word's meaning appears as a feeling.[14] P. Janet described a patient of his who stood for 48 hours on her toes in front of an imaginary crucifix, with stigmatic hemorrhaging from her wrists and feet in the places where nails were driven in when crucifying.[183]

When searching for the neurobiological basis of mystical and spiritual practices, increased activity in the frontal and temporal lobes of the brain is found, in addition to increased serotonin and dopaminergic activity.[31] LSD, which stimulates serotonin activity and causes mystical experiences, and cocaine, which increases dopamine activity, particularly in the nucleus accumbens, have similar effects. Increased activity in the temporal lobe and the limbic system is also present when paranormal beliefs, delusions, and hallucinations are combined with hyper-religious content (like being raped by the devil, or impregnated by a saint), which provides evidence for the hypothesis that temporo-limbic dysfunction is a common neuronal substrate for mediating both hyper-religiosity and psychotic experiences.[31, 120]

The idiosyncratic varieties of faith in closed communities like heresies or sects may result in tragedy. The founder or leader of most sects is frequently a well-functioning charismatic male individual suffering from mental illness, usually paranoid psychosis (most frequently a paraphrenic one) without negative symptoms, and displays a contagious emotionality, as well as good communicative and manipulative skills. Regardless of the variations in subject matter of the delusional content, this charismatic leader's main message is his special connection to God, or that he *is* God (theomegalomania). As the cult's leader, he requires, as a rule, unconditional obedience. Jim Jones of Guyana forcing 900 members to drink poison in order to be transferred to another planet is just one example.

Healthy religious feelings are based on the harmony between self-assertion and self-devotion, and do not go to extremes.[161] The cult of suffering in some closed and fundamentalist Christian denominations has resulted in members' withdrawal from secularity and civilizational achievements, rejecting any and all pleasures, and self-inflicting harm. In Bulgaria, one such teaching is found in Hesychasm (meaning "staying in silence", due to their vow of silence), and another, to a certain extent, in the Danov School which was founded several centuries later. The mass castrations performed in the so-called sect of castrates in Russia during the 18th and 19th centuries, as well as the castration of young boys in Catholic choruses for the purpose of preserving the high timbre of their voices, are well known. Intense, compulsive reading of the Bible, sometimes until loss of consciousness, and altering one's appearance with haircuts or wearing strange clothing are signs of a severe risk for autoaggression.[121] The advice in Matthew's gospel not to marry, but live as a eunuch if possible (Matthew 19: 11–12), as well as Jesus' message that anyone who looks at a woman with lust has already committed adultery, with the advice to gauge out one's eye and cut one's hand if they cause one to falter (Matthew 5: 28–33), could be accepted as literal, and have been the basis for not a small number of psychotic self-mutilations.

Clinical case. A 48-year-old man, with an onset of illness 25 years before, who prayed round-the-clock, secluded himself, defecated in his room, banged his forehead against the floor in a stereotypical fashion, and heard voices accusing him of sins and demanding redemption. He did not allow his room to be cleaned and did not cut his hair, shave, or trim his nails for years due to his being "undeserving". Despite neuroleptic treatment, at the age of 38 he gauged out his both eyes with a knife under the influence of voices which accused him of having lustful thoughts about his brother's wife. The enucleation was done in cold blood, with the consecutive removal ("first the right one, which was the first to sin, then the left...") of the eyeballs and absence of shock due to pain or blood loss. The patient shared that he had not, in fact, had such thoughts, but had instead contemplated whether or not they were feasible as a challenge, or "suggestion" from his sister-in-law, while the voices hinted that such contemplation was equivalent to experiencing the act. For 10 years afterwards, he was on continuous antipsychotic treatment, learned Braille, and worked from his home as a translator; and the hallucinosis became chronic, with decreasing intensity and isolated exacerbations with insomnia, an influx of ideas about sin and redemption, and accusatory "satanic" voices. At the age of 48 he committed suicide, and was discovered with many cutting wounds on his genitalia and chest.

Like in many schizophrenia onsets, the patient's behavior at the beginning of the psychosis resembled a hermit's seclusion. Religious toxicity, however, only added content and additional motivation to the pathological phenomena—negative symptoms, verbal hallucinations, delusions, first-rank symptoms in paralogical relatedness (the thought of something turns it into a reality)—and influenced the patient's behavior in an imperative manner. Brutal auto-mutilations are characteristic of schizophrenia. What was particularly startling in this case was the anesthesia during self-enucleation, probably affectively determined, similarly to mystical states with narrowed consciousness. Delusions and hallucinations with religious content are some of the longest enduring ones in clinical practice. Many other delusional subject matters may change with time, but the topic of religion, just like hypochondria and jealousy, is steady as a rule—and with its lack of alternatives, it does not allow for convincing distinctions to be made between its delusional and overvalued qualities, despite clinical improvement. As in roughly half of all patients with schizophrenia (Chapter 8), decades after the severe onset, clinical stabilization and even improvement in functioning, within the limitations of deficits, were achieved. Regardless of improvement, however, the fatal end came about in a brutal and uncompromising way, leaving no doubt, with the wounds found on the genitalia, about the patient's psychotic religious motivation, so closely mirroring his act of enucleation 10 years earlier.

Clinical case. A 59-year-old patient, whose mother, ex-wife, and son were all diagnosed with schizophrenia, experienced nocturnal enuresis until the age of 10 and became interested in religion and philosophy during his teen years, later becoming a convinced believer. At the same time, after hearing a remark that he was fat, he reduced his eating, started counting calories, and vomiting, losing 15 kg. During regular military service, he made an attempt to poison himself with medications prescribed for "neurotic" problems, and was dismissed. Graduating with a degree in theology, he got a job as a maintenance worker in a local bishop's residence, where he still remains at present. He started visiting different specialists and ordering a lot of laboratory tests due to his suspicion that he was being poisoned, and monitoring habitual activities, e.g., eating with a spoon, due to his feeling that they had lost their automaticity and were in need of control.

During the schism of the Bulgarian Orthodox Church in the early 90s, he claimed that it was caused by the Korean religious leader Moon and his wife, showing a photo of Mrs. Moon where the image of Satan could be recognized. He burned banknotes because he saw the devil on them, but since the devil did not exist (according to Saint Augustine), believed the image had been a sign that the notes had no effect. Seized by the fear that some crimes would be imputed to him, he walked barefooted, undressed and whipped himself on his father's grave, sensed that his jacket was emitting signals, heard voices discussing him, and thought that he was being secretly surveilled and influenced in peculiar ways, including through the appearance of corns on his feet while he was smoking. He felt guilty about the lack of snow in the winter because he had profaned nature by masturbating in the mountains. He made a suicide attempt by suffocating himself and, when he failed, asked his mother to finish him.

Since this overt episode which led to his first hospitalization, the patient has been on regular maintenance treatment. He met his future wife during one of his hospital stays: they married and had a child, and after their divorce and her detainment in a chronic psychiatric hospital, he cares for his son alone, and adequately so. The episodes which followed featured delusions with similar content, but less intensity, and between episodes he did sustain some strange beliefs, e.g., continuing to think that the image of Satan on banknotes is a well-kept financial secret, and still has fluctuating self-reference ideas. After 35 years, however, he continues to work in the same place, enjoys reading books, maintains the household, and has adequate concern for his son due to the family history of schizophrenia on both parents' sides. Aware of the high genetic risk, he took him for prophylactic visits to a psychiatrist even before the boy's illness onset.

This story illustrates parallel trajectories of illness and religiosity. Although religious themes are interpolated within the psychotic content, especially during the full-blown episode with bizarre, grandiose delusions, his job in the bishop's residence and practicing of religious rituals do not extend beyond what is commonplace and conventionally accepted. Despite unfavorable factors such as heredity, prodrome anorexia (usually a precursor to schizophrenia in boys, and affective disorders in girls when not genuine anorexia nervosa), manifestations resembling neurosis, and depersonalization, the subsequent course has been a favorable one. His desire to have a family and children, even from a mentally ill mother, adequate parental role, continuous employment in a milieu which is in unison with his faith, available support and tolerance (the priests encourage him to maintain contact with psychiatric services), good insight and treatment compliance, as well as non-doctrinal religiosity in the framework of a large, normative religion (*mainstream* Orthodox Christianity) rather than in a sect or cult all contribute to the favorable course. Religiosity in this case has had a benevolent impact on his illness behavior and compliance with treatment. True religiosity usually leads to humility and accepting the need for treatment as a duty, while sect doctrines may suggest the rejection of mental health services, instead subjecting believers to exorcism or other magical methods that bear a closer resemblance to paranormal practices.

Clinical case. A 33-year old-Arab, living with his parents and brothers in the country for several years, was hospitalized several times for hearing voices with unpleasant and sometimes blasphemous content and sudden alterations in motor behavior: suddenly stopping in the middle of the street, rushing, or rolling on the ground—something particularly dangerous when in public places. During one of his hospitalizations he stripped naked, dusted his body with antiperspirant powder, and, yelling "Allahu akbar", smashed the mounted TV set in the foyer of the ward with a chair. After getting his excitement under control, he insisted on being punished. Since then, he has been on clozapine and has not been admitted again for years, but is passive, displays vague tension, with inserted thoughts acquiring sound qualities during exacerbations, and is tormented by obsessions with a blasphemous character making him pray.

In this clinical picture, a pathoplasticity of cultural transition can be noticed over the religious content of the patient's hallucinations and delusions. Blasphemy, redemption, and obsessive doubts are all traits of a Christian mentality, as well as being significant themes in psychosis, depression, and obsessive-compulsive disorder. They are uncommon in Islam. Direct communication with God, or with the Prophet, is not distinctive of traditional Islam, and any attempt to attribute human qualities to them (or even portray them), or make them subject to doubt or indecent attitudes, is so obscene that the taboo is not disturbed even in psychosis. The patient's family is from a secular environment in the Muslim country of their origin, and is well adapted in their new residence, where they continue to ritually maintain their traditions, however without much zeal. The "Europeanization" of his symptomatology with blasphemous and obsessive elements enter into such conflict, however, with taboos regarding the Prophet that the patient describes his experiences in a roundabout way, without mentioning the name. The illness' cultural cleavage lies between a Christian pattern of phenomena and his horror at their incompatibility with what is most sacred in Islam. Small doses of antidepressant improved the obsessive phenomena (likely also facilitated by clozapine). At the same time, his illness behavior is dominated by trends characteristic of his traditional background: he will not start working until he has "gotten well", and experiences shame about being unmarried. The cultural matrix and pathoplasticity of religious content in his psychosis combine with one another in a way which demonstrates the need for sensitive assessment of individual culture, and cautions against stereotypes.

6.2 The Paranormal and Psychopathology

As pointed out, the paranormal satisfies more the need to protect oneself against basic anxiety, and find solutions through miracles, than the need for meaning and consolation which is more characteristic of religiosity. As contrasted to paranormal belief, paranormal experience is a first-hand sensation, e.g., the direct feeling of aliens' influence. It is usually regarded as abnormal even by representatives of the subculture sharing the same beliefs. This distinction has its analogue in religiosity too: faith in God is praiseworthy, while direct communication with Him is not encouraged, and can be considered sinful and condemnable.[73, 161]

Magic beliefs and practices manifest differently depending on the current topical superstitions—from burning witches in the Middle Ages to contemporary esoteric cults, telepathy, and extra-sensory effects. Scientific development has not substantially altered the need for miracles, but only shapes such manifestations accordingly: energy fields, poltergeists, aliens, psychotronic weapons, etc. People differ in the degree of their maturity about and susceptibility to magical thinking. There is a link between paranormal beliefs and histories of childhood trauma in the general population, as well as among the mentally ill.[176] Crises and illnesses usually mobilize one's aptitude for paranormal beliefs through sparing the burden of personal responsibility. The fact that misfortunes, over which one has no power, can be more easily endured this way explains why suffering is the most fertile ground for growing magic beliefs.

Paranormal explanatory schemes are varied, e.g., the roles of magnetic storms in changing blood pressure, the evil eye's responsibility for nocturnal enuresis, negative energies, karma, and extra-sensory abilities having their effects on one's personal fate, including states of health and illness. The mothers of dehydrated children in the Third World frequently refuse oral rehydration because of the belief that diarrhea is caused by magic.[84] The subject matters of magic which appear to have a touch of science do not alter the magic's essence. The attribution of unclear symptoms, like feebleness or a bad mood, to viruses, gases, or categories like chronic fatigue syndrome is, in general, not very different from referring to magic. Contemporary "mass hysteria", e.g., as described in young girls presenting symptoms of intoxication by industrial agents (unconfirmed after thorough examination), has the mechanism of its rise in common with the medieval resurgence of epidemics.[218] Bulgaria's traditional cultural notion that the common cold is the cause of many diseases exemplifies a likely explanation being used to satisfy the human need for clarity. In contemporary medicine, the linear causal paradigm is only partially relevant to infectious and, in some rare cases, genetic diseases, while the etiopathogenesis of other diseases can be expressed mainly in terms of their diathesis, statistical likelihood, and multiple other factors—in opposition to the mass need for simpler explanations. As noted by S. Freud, believing in chance requires certain intellectual training, as the primitive, uneducated, or childlike will find some reason in everything that happens, e.g., to them, everybody dies due to someone else's fault (usually the doctor's).[62]

The ideological conflict between the representatives of official medicine and paranormal subculture is, to a certain extent, due to the pathologization of magical beliefs. An extreme form of this view is the vulgarization that all magical aberrations are symptoms of mental disorder. Undoubtedly, personality abnormalities, traumatic experiences, and unsolved inner conflicts predispose people to belief in superstitions; however, the mechanisms by which superstitions cope with problems are no different from other known defense mechanisms. Equating the paranormal with mental illness rests on a reductionistic categorization of the unintelligible—this is in fact similar to the function carried out by magic belief itself, i.e., reducing what is unacceptable down to a plain scheme devised by an external power.

Although paranormal beliefs have been the subject of many studies, their specific relationship with psychopathology remains unclear. Most data in this area are epidemiological, and show a high prevalence rate: in Greece, 85 % of psychotic patients' mothers attribute the state of their children to magic,[216] and in Malawi, 53 % of all psychiatric patients attribute their illness to witches and evil spirits.[170] Delusional processing of magical stories from folklore is particularly frequent among Indian[127, 128] and South African patients.[204] Also found in high frequency is the belief in demonic causes for illness among schizophrenic patients (56 %), as well as in nonpsychotic ones, though to a lesser degree.[162] Analysis of the delusional content in 200 patients with schizophrenia in the South African Xhosa tribe finds that 72.5 % of think that their illness is because of magic as a result of their envy or jealousy—taking into account the fact that belief in such magic is also common among healthy persons from the same tribe.[34] There is an association between magic beliefs, lower levels of education, and rural origins, and a Pakistani study shows the possibility of deducing delusional content in schizophrenic patients based on socio-cultural factors, with topics associated with black magic being more frequent in impoverished female patients.[201] The role of local explanations and norms for tolerance towards odd behaviors is accepted as the leading precedent for discriminating between delusional and non-delusional magical thinking.[2, 65]

The link between paranormal beliefs and experiences and psychosis is twofold: the paranormal may be either an inducing factor or the product of psychosis.

The role of the paranormal in inducing psychoses is usually regarded as a precipitating but not etiological one.[161, 186] The emergence of mental disorder in persons who are dedicated to mystical and esoteric practices is commonly attributed to their underlying vulnerability. According to some evidence, the frequency of mental illness among the members of sects does not vary much from that in the general population,[66] and the state of some patients with schizophrenia is even stabilized when joining sects and cults.

There are, however, some induced dissociative states with altered consciousness, motorics, and identity,[54, 70, 75, 153, 186] presenting first-rank symptoms, whose main characteristics include preceding auto-induction and an impression of playfulness and imitation. Their analysis demonstrates that transcendent experiences can cause psychosis, not to mention that psychogenesis cannot be reduced to psychotrauma alone, but is also associated with desirable, even pleasurable experiences like voluntarily immersing oneself in mysticism. For this reason, contemporary models of reactive psychosis replace *psychotrauma* with *life events*, and *psychogenesis* (which only accounts for its psychogenic influence) with *reactivity* (accounting for the interaction of psychogenic influence with vulnerability and predisposition).[45, 144, 163] The nosological status of reactive psychosis remains, however, questionable due to uncertainty about favorable outcome being a validating principle, as well as the lack of diagnostic stability over time. Nevertheless, the presence of Schneider's first-rank phenomena in psychosis induced by paranormal experiences suggests that their presence in reactive states is also feasible.[159]

Evidently, the dissociative mechanism in the genesis of self-disturbance in psychosis is a universal one, and the division between the endogenous and psychogenic is relative. The dissociative model schematizes a separation of the conscious from the unconscious, as well as of different mental functions from one another. Although the sources for this model are mainly hysteria, hypnotical phenomena, and multiple personalities, the mechanism of dissociation itself—briefly defined as the psyche's weakened capacity for synthesis[182]—is common to the basic disturbances in schizophrenia, i.e., splitting of functions, going as far as the fragmentation of one's mental life. This is by no means astonishing: historically, dissociation has been the original model, from which Bleuler developed his concept of schizophrenia,[182] described in the modern neuroscientific context as a *weakness of brain links* or *cognitive dysmetria*.[9] Pathogenesis of psychosis induced by paranormal themes includes a targeted affinity of the paranormal for dissociation—because of its tendency to separate, (initially in self-defense), certain psychological functions, traumatic experiences, and aspects of self-knowledge and self-control. Herein lies the phenomenological similarity between dissociation and first-rank symptoms: a pathological loss of autonomous mental functions, which induces self-disturbance in both dissociative disorders and schizophrenia.

The examination of paranormal beliefs and experiences, not just as precursors to but also as products of psychosis, finds its adequate interpretation only through differentiating between symptom form and content. This differentiation was made clear in the first place by Jaspers.[104] The symptom's *form* determines the nature of a pathological phenomenon and its assignment to a certain category of psychopathology, e.g., an overvalued idea, an obsession, or a delusion, while the symptom's *content* is the specific subject matter which fills it. Until the 19th century, physicians had failed to develop a comparative psychopathology, for the most part because the content of symptoms, rather than their form, was scrutinized.[210] The paranormal is most frequently evoked as an explanatory topic belonging to symptom content. This belonging has been well conceptualized in theories of attribution style in delusion formation, cognitive deficits, defense mechanisms of delusions, and the vulnerability-stress model in psychosis.[129] The paranormal also plays a pathoplastic role in psychosis, subordinating illness behavior to the theme of abnormal experiences.

Delusional mood and psychotic anticipations of large-scale catastrophes are experiences without trivial analogues or credible explanations. Conversion to the paranormal introduces order, calm, and even a feeling of personal importance. In such cases, paranormal beliefs and experiences are secondary to psychosis, and may have some defensive function. Signs which can tell apart mentally ill mystics from healthy ones are neither related to the content of their beliefs and practices (they may be identical) nor the generally accepted criteria for psychosis: both may have experiences which contradict empirical testing and are not accessible for feedback and correction through arguments or evidence. What remains crucial for such distinctions to be made are the accompanying features of dysfunction in mental illness: the inability to control one's entry into odd states, or their duration, the deterioration of habits, and neglecting everyday ritual obligations that have cultural congruence.[73]

The practice of psychiatry in Bulgaria also has its traditions and has made contributions to the complex scope of paranormal themes interplaying with psychopathology: analyses of states observed in Pentecostals[161] and fire walkers (*nestinari*)[186] (presented along with spirit possession states[153] and *extra sense* psychoses in Chapter 7), the iatrogenic influence of religion and magic, including the mechanism of so-called voodoo death—caused by a curse where an ossicle is pointed at the victim, and which can be prevented only by counter-magic,[183] and the impact of beliefs in magic and aliens on the delusional content described by a large sample of psychotic patients.[156]

In a study of 711 patients with schizophrenia, schizoaffective, and bipolar affective disorder (BAD) in Bulgaria, we assessed the content of delusions where beliefs in magic and aliens were present, as well as their correlation with clinical sociodemographic factors.[156] Religious delusions were excluded from the focus of the study, due to their conceptual distinction from the paranormal dimension, especially with monotheism. After content analysis of data from records and interviews with the Schedules for Clinical Assessment in Neuropsychiatry (SCAN), such beliefs were identified in 19.8 % of all patients: 10.4 % with beliefs in magic and 10.1 % with beliefs in aliens, and an insignificant overlap between them.

The experiences associated with magic were divided into the following categories: magic beliefs—purely thought phenomena; magic rituals—behaviors related to beliefs; objectivized magic—identification of magic with specific material objects, e.g., a lock of hair, a stone, or animal fur; and the involvement of a relative in some magical subject matter. Examples of magic beliefs might include the conviction that one has been bewitched by a fortune-teller, being empowered by "white" magic to fight evil forces, or being under a spell which causes eternal suffering. Some magic rituals are actions for preventing or undoing magic, such as taking a shower fully clothed so that the magic cannot penetrate through the water, killing cats or frogs, avoiding certain people, food, or clothes because they are bewitched, visiting an imam to undo magic, and—in cases of objectivized magic—excessive cleansing for the purposes of removing magical agents, e.g., hair, animal feces, suspicious cups of coffee or glasses of water, or unusually placed toys or clothes.

Typical examples of beliefs in aliens include hearing voices, communicating with them via telepathy, and experiencing thought insertion, possession, or abduction by aliens. It is apparent that, while magic beliefs and rituals in the psychotic experience do resemble superstitions incidental to the subculture and are even shared by some healthy persons from the same population, beliefs in aliens manifest themselves within the structure of frankly abnormal experiences, in most cases as the subject matter of first-rank symptoms.

Beliefs in magic are twice as common in women, while beliefs in aliens are almost equally present in both men and women. There is a trending two-to-three-fold increase in the frequencies of both kinds of beliefs following the transition of diagnosis from BAD, through schizophrenia, to schizoaffective disorder. No association was found between the frequency of these beliefs and patients' education or grades in school. Only 25.7 % of patients believing in magic during an illness episode ever expressed such beliefs out of psychosis, i.e., before the psychosis onset or during remission; and none of the patients believing in aliens ever shared such beliefs outside of an illness episode.

These results show a lower prevalence of believing in magic among psychotic patients than might be expected, according to their distribution in the general population. A public poll in the country with a representative sample of 1000 individuals over 15 years of age found that half of respondents believed in telepathy and clairvoyance, around 60 % believed they could be easily placed under a spell, and approximately every fifth person was aware of specific instances of "black" or "white" magic.[156] It is unclear whether these responses reflect their true beliefs, and how they relate to patient beliefs from our sample. It is usually assumed that symptom content in psychopathology reflects subcultural beliefs. The low prevalence of those believing in magic and the absence of believers in aliens *outside* of illness in this sample demonstrates, however, that the beliefs *during* illness are a product of the psychosis, rather than an illness extension of paranormal subcultural beliefs. It turns out that paranormal beliefs in the general population and among psychiatric patients are separate phenomena, not a continuum—in contrast with the prevailing view in transcultural psychiatry. This interpretation is also supported by the fact that the frequency of beliefs in magic and aliens within the sample group demonstrated no correlations to sociodemographic variables; it did, however, depend strongly on the diagnosis—with differences up to three-fold in frequency between diagnostic categories.

Assessment of the associations between these beliefs and some clinical characteristics in the schizophrenia group within the sample finds a negative correlation between beliefs in magic and the quality of remission, age at illness onset, presence of formal thought disorder, and number of hospitalizations. This negative association with these variables demonstrates a more favorable course of illness and may be related to a certain protective function of magic beliefs in psychosis. The cultural role of magic is to oppress contradictions between what the ideal world should be and what it is in reality.[43] The protective role of paranormal beliefs in psychosis shows that, although magic beliefs in health and psychosis are separate entities (and not a common dimension), their defense functions seem to be similar.

From an anthropological viewpoint, magic beliefs flourish in communities where the generally accepted social stance regarding conflict resolution is lacking, and childhood aggression and sexuality provoke intense anxiety.[43] Two main mechanisms by which magic exerts its influence are described: imitation, i.e., actions similar to the intended result, and contagiousness, i.e., physical touch as an extension of spiritual contact.[198] Imitation is similar to magic rituals from our categorization; contagiousness—to objectivized magic.

The collision between paranormal beliefs and scientific medicine is, in essence, a cultural collision. Paranormal expressiveness in suffering is frantic and irrational, often masked as an appeal for help or exaggeration, while medical practitioners are usually technocratic and skeptical, and the superstitious performance most frequently arouses undisguised irritation. The path to effective help does not pass through confrontation and sarcasm, nor through the condemnation of beliefs,[217] but it does come with the clear message that sharing a common view about the world is not necessary for either giving or receiving help. A serious barrier in front of this dialog is dogmatism. The medical profession is a privileged subculture in every society,[84] and, as such, physicians are used to being accepted as the carriers of valid truths in their field. Intervening in cases with paranormal experiences is imperative for certain mental disorders, whose characteristics should be determined by the nature of the disorder, not its subject matter. Dynamics in the families of victims of sects is also a domain of assistance, and the therapeutic principles applied to patients' recovery after paranormal intoxication closely resemble such approaches used in treating former captives, victims of disasters, and survivors after torture or loss—facilitating the processing of grief and reintegration.

7 Spirit Possession States

The Devil inside us (İçimizdeki Şeytan).

S. Ali

The experience of possession by spirits or other supernatural forces is part of the heritage of different civilizations and is rooted in numerous religious traditions and cults. It occurs in various states, and explanations for it vacillate between hysteria, charlatanism, schizophrenia, and "brainwashing". These conditions are integral to the interweaving of cultural models and psychopathology, and their interpretation is a test for hypotheses in this area. Such interweaving and its interpretation are illustrated here through the analysis of clinical cases from two very different cultures: Swahili and Bulgarian.

Possession states are a challenge to clinical psychiatry. First of all, the distinction between normative and pathological possession remains vague. Besides, the pathological type's nosological status is also unclear. These states are usually conceptualized as unique culture-specific syndromes or as varieties of dissociative disorders. In the latter case, possession experience in the Third World is pointed out as analogous to multiple personality disorder in developed countries.[188] Claims that these states represent a separate clinical entity[1] appear debatable in the context of a two-year follow up of patients with dissociative disorders in India which does not identify dissociative sub-categories related to identity disturbances, trance, and possession.[3] This is similar to the situation of possession's Western "twin", multiple personality disorder:[134] while some doubt its existence in general, accusing media and psychoanalytical culture of stimulating behaviors that resemble identity change,[188] others recognize it frequently and even recommend its routine assessment.[176] The questions outnumber the answers: how are normative and pathological possession experiences differentiated? How is behavior in distress shaped by local beliefs about possession? Are possession experiences symptoms of specific syndromes or manifestations of known mental disorders? Clinical analysis of cases from a traditional culture where possession states are unusually common may offer some of the answers to these questions.

7.1 Clinical Cases from Pemba Island

Traditions in Pemba Island are relevant to these issues because of the special status the island holds in Swahili culture: it was believed for centuries to be the center of witchcraft in East Africa. Pemba is the second largest island of Zanzibar, part of Tanzania since 1964. It is situated some 40 miles from the East African coast, just south of the Equator. The island's history is filled with stories about early seafaring trips made by the Shirazi (people of Persian origin) with dhows and the mythical Sinbad; this history also includes centuries-long Arab hegemony, Portuguese and British domination, and affluence under the Omani Sultanate in the 19th and 20th centuries, during which Zanzibar was for decades the capital of East Africa and the southern part of the Arabian Peninsula.

Both verbal and written ancient stories were strongly influenced by beliefs in spirits of various origins; these have directly shaped Swahili identity. Archaic pagan cults (*kafiri*) were blended with those from the Islamic tradition (*kiislamu*), spirits from the mainland (*bara*) were mixed with coastal ones (*pwani*), and local spirits (*kipemba*) were combined with foreign elements (*kigala, kizungu, kiarabu,* etc.). The resulting mixture is unique for the Swahili cosmogony. Beliefs in spirits are still widespread and a part of everyday life. Many residents have their own "personal" spirits which are usually benevolent (*jinni*), haunting the bushes around the huts from where they are called on to cope with problems, illnesses or some other misfortunes. Local masters of magic (*watchawi*) have control over black magic (*juju*) and evil spirits (*shetani*), but also over the art of healing by means of magic. Considered to be the most powerful practitioners of witchcraft in East Africa, their "headquarters" are located in South Pemba. I observed the clinical cases described below between 1996 and 1998 at Chake-Chake Hospital on the island.

Clinical case. A 29-year-old female patient, married with four children, comes to the out-patient clinic with complaints of total and unbearable possession by an evil spirit (*shetani*) which forces her to undress, yell, pace around the family's hut, and experience anguish and "stupidity". Although well-formulated, the commands are not described as voices, but rather as irresistible thoughts from her inner world—dominated by *shetani*. Clinical examination finds perplexity and chaotic behavior ("I am forced to act foolishly… there is no sense whatsoever; I am a stupid woman… I happen to put sand in the food and I do not know why…"), as well as agitation, tenseness, lack of hope for improvement, and a self-denigrating attitude. Her possession was preceded by unclear discomfort and an inability to experience pleasure.

Some difficulties in this case stem from the focus on the possession experience in the patient's rapport and the lack of a genuine low mood. Verbalization of possession claims, however, is of help when making a precise clinical assessment. The patient's inability to clearly trace the origin of the commands (from her inner world that is, in turn, dominated by *shetani*) and her absolute obedience to an external force could easily be misinterpreted as first-rank symptoms. The diagnosis of depression is confirmed by the course of the episode: vague complaints with a lack of pleasure at the beginning, followed by an inability to cope with everyday life, and, subsequently, a possession experience as the explanation for the preceding tormenting symptoms. In this context, the command automatism is a mood-congruent, pseudo-first-rank phenomenon. This was confirmed by the patient's good response and complete recovery following a 4-week treatment with amitriptyline. Formally, her condition meets the criteria for psychotic depression because of her firm belief in spirits. In her disorganized behavior, however, elements of a dissociative narrowing of consciousness were evident, and the improvement was too rapid—without any need to increase the antidepressant dose or introduce an antipsychotic.

Clinical case. A 50-year-old married female seeks help with an unbearable sense of being possessed by *shetani* which makes her brood, shout at her grandchild, and pour water on her head. She complains, "That child drives me crazy with crying, I'll throw her out…Sometimes I mix fish with sand, and I shout and run and run until I collapse from exhaustion and find a place to rest…" During the interview there are visible autonomous symptoms, muscle tension, an inability to relax, frequent sighing and persistent ruminative worries, partial amnesia after excessive shouting, and fears about possible diseases caused by *shetani*. Careful clarification reveals that she does not literally experience possession, but presumes it because of the "futility" of her actions. She seems willing to accept another explanation for her condition, for instance a medical one, if it would help her to overcome it. It becomes apparent that she had similar complaints 30 years ago when recovering after the treatment of a traditional healer (*mganga*), while the current episode began approximately a year ago and has not so far been improved by traditional or magic healers (*watchawi*).

The clinical picture in this case meets the criteria for generalized anxiety disorder. The diagnostic difficulties are shaped by the subjective incomprehensibility of the experience and the patient's inability to connect her complaints to people or events from her surroundings that would make sense of them. No other explanation for this unintelligible experience, apart from the belief in being possessed, is available in her personal background and her milieu. The belief in being possessed by an evil spirit (*shetani*) adds drama to the behavior, serves as a convenient explanatory matrix, and is easily reinforced by previous experience. In this case, anxiety with accompanying autonomous phenomena are directly experienced, while possession is a subsequent explanation (i.e., ideatory phenomenon) but not a direct experience.

Clinical case. An 18-year-old female, unmarried, attempted to run away from her home because an evil spirit had made her vulnerable to two of her neighbors who wanted to slay her. The behavioral change started with gloominess and several days' withdrawal, escalating to tension, insomnia, and violence. She yelled at her relatives to stay away from her because a devil had taken control of her brain and she could no longer command her own actions and wishes. During the clinical examination, she shares that a devil sends her orders and "opens" her mind to the two neighbors who want to kill her as revenge for an alleged past insult. She is certain that the devil is making her hear the voices of her neighbors in order to torment her.

Evident upon examination are command automatism with thought broadcasting, commenting and third-person verbal hallucinations, delusions of possession and imminent destruction, and risky psychotic behavior. The possession experience encompasses both symptom content and her relatives' explanations of the illness. Her state meets the criteria for an acute schizophreniform episode (with the duration criterion for schizophrenia, though most likely onset, not being met). For local people in such cases, being *possessed* is literally equivalent to being *ill*. First, others sought help from a "witch doctor" (*watchawi*) but the patient physically attacked him, convinced that he was possessed by an evil spirit. Then she was urgently brought to the psychiatric outpatient unit. Treatment with haloperidol led to a complete recovery in two weeks. Despite the acuteness of the patient's symptoms, and the fact that the treatment response was good, the prognosis remains cautious.

Clinical case. A 26-year-old single male complains of discomfort and a crawling sensation on his skin and head, accompanied by an unpleasant cracking. The patient is certain that this has been caused by a spirit as a warning of the imminent destruction of his brain. According to him, the spirit is being commanded from a distance by evil *watchawi* via black magic. His interview reveals insomnia and loss of appetite, energy, and interest in pleasant experiences. His brother and sister are mentally ill.

The patient's explanatory scheme introduces paranoid elements, as well as the probable diagnostic confusion of a clinical picture that meets the criteria for psychotic depression. In Muslim populations, "endogenous" depression may lack feelings of guilt and low moods at the expense of somatic signs.[78] In this case, reduced energy, a lack of appetite, anhedonia, somatic and simple auditory hallucinations, and, congruent with the total experience, delusional interpretations are evident.

Clinical case. A 19-year-old single male with a history of grand-mal seizures starting in childhood complains that his personal spirit, called Dodoo—benevolent until recently—has started to torment him. The episodes always precede seizures which last for half an hour and follow a common sequence: Dodoo directly enters the body and self of the patient, who experiences increasing bodily aches, detachment from his surroundings, loss of hearing, and a state of bewilderment in which the patient and Dodoo are indistinguishable, followed by a loss of consciousness and grand-mal type seizure. Upon awakening, he feels better, oriented, and hungry. An old EEG record made on the mainland shows signs of temporal lobe epilepsy.

Despite the lack of an EEG machine on the island, the diagnosis of epilepsy does not cause particular doubt. The possession experience followed imminently by a seizure does shape a peculiar *possession aura*. The mystical content, reflecting the ancient "sacred illness", illustrates the nosological variety of possession states. Adjusting the dose of phenytoin, which the patient had been taking for a long time, decreases the frequency of the seizures and of Dodoo's preceding intrusions.

Clinical case. A 32-year-old married female with two children is afraid that she has been the victim of witchcraft for three months because of sudden possessions by a spirit which last for about 20 minutes nearly every day, sometimes several times a day. During these episodes, she experiences strong fear for her safety and sanity. She also sweats, feels heaviness in her chest, has difficulty breathing, and feels faint—there have been a couple of real collapses, though she has not hurt herself. There are no complaints apart from the episodes, with the exception of mild lassitude and concern about these anticipated "moments of terror".

The diagnosis of panic disorder is apparent from the key features of the clinical picture. Periodic possession here is tautological to periodic anxiety, while attribution to magic is a secondary interpretation. Despite a positive response to the prescribed antidepressant, the patient soon stopped taking it under the influence of her relatives, the symptoms recurred, and she started visiting local healers.

These case records are loose descriptions, not systematically collected data. The structured assessment of psychopathology, however, is problematic in traditional cultures. Structured clinical instruments are the product of research paradigms in developed countries, and their cultural applicability outside these countries is unknown, while the conversational context of the interviews is not very typical for cultures with a collective hegemony.[134, 150] In such communities, idiosyncratic descriptions and so-called quality research based approaches are more relevant for grasping unique experiences than the more structured instruments that extract nomothetic, "digital" types of data.

The implications of the cases described above can be viewed on several levels: normative possession beliefs, delineation between form and content of symptoms, links between symptoms and their impact on functioning, and nosological heterogeneity of the clinical states. *Normative* possession beliefs in Pemba are rooted in Swahili cosmology and are reinforced by collective traditions. They are devoid of the metaphysical attributes present in similar beliefs held by Medieval Europeans, and are instead trivialized to everyday functions. They fulfill basic human needs such as survival and acceptance by others and, explicably, are mobilized in times of distress. The attribution of misfortunes to evil spirits (*shetani*) or black magic (*juju*) conjured by magicians (*watchawi*) is analogous to intrapsychic defense mechanisms, as they serve the same purposes. What is conventional in one culture may appear paranormal in another.[175] Where collective values dominate above individual ones, attributing one's misfortunes to external forces can have a relieving effect on suffering through the denouncement personal responsibility. Projecting such intelligibility from normal to pathological possession, however, should be done cautiously.

Much misunderstanding that concerns possession states derives from nondistinction between the form and content of symptoms (Chapter 6). Morbid contents change over time. European "demon possessions" and "witch mania" in the 17th century gave way to modern "intoxications" by viruses and gases, but the mechanisms of symptom production have remained very much the same—as if to remind us that education and science do not protect us from our own gullibility.[218] In the described cases, the experiences of being possessed by spirits clearly belong to the symptoms' content, while the symptom complex is different in each case. In the literature, two main tendencies may be outlined in the interpretation of possession experiences: either as the content of symptoms in delusions[71, 95] and dissociative disorders[22, 54] or as culture-bound states that cannot be reduced to other common clinical syndromes.[1, 28, 75] The latter approach is problematic in its validating criteria, including treatment and outcome. Indicative of this is the failure of exorcism treatment in cases of "ghost possession" which only remitted after "Western diagnoses" were accepted and relevant neuroleptic treatment was provided.[77]

What remains crucial for diagnosis (and, hence, for treatment) in these cases are not the possession experiences themselves, but the symptom context in which they are manifested, as well as the accompanying features of dysfunction. The main diagnostic difficulties are due to the pathoplastic influence of symptom content on symptom form (in the sense of Jaspers). Part of what is called "culture-bound" in psychiatry refers to the specific contents of otherwise known clinical states. Dramatic as they are, possession experiences may blur other signs of the clinical picture, like anhedonia and loss of libido or appetite, without which the correct diagnosis (depression) may be missed. The golden rule in the diagnostic process is to always account for the whole symptom complex, not just for the symptom content. Assessing concomitant features of dysfunction is also essential, particularly in cases where delineating between normative and pathological beliefs and experiences proves difficult. In specific subcultures, the deterioration of day-to-day functioning and self-control during psychosis—but not the possession experience per se—are perceived as pathological by others and are the reason to seek out psychiatric treatment.[73] In possession disorder with a dissociative nature, on the other hand, most patients manage to maintain normal social functioning in spite of their claims of demonic possession.[54]

The case records from Pemba Island, a culture with rich traditions in magic and mass spirit beliefs, show nosological heterogeneity of possession experiences. Among the prototypic cases in the ICD-10 Casebook,[212] possession is described in one case with severe depression and in another with dissociative (trance and possession) disorder. There is already sufficient consensus that possession states should be identified as dissociative disorders. The cases described here, however, demonstrate much broader heterogeneity: depression, anxiety disorders, schizophreniform psychosis, and epilepsy.

7.2 Bulgarian Analogues of Possession

The clinical descriptions of mystical states with possession in Pentecostals[161] and in fire dancers or *nestinari*[186] are part of the classic Bulgarian psychiatric legacy. Similar phenomena found later on have included the so-called extra sense psychoses during the 1990s. Unjustly forgotten, the Bulgarian psychiatrist Dr. Hristo Petrov (Fig. 8)—killed in Alexandrovska Hospital on January 10, 1944, during the bombing of Sofia—described glossolalia among Pentecostals in his study "Psychology and psychopathology of the religious feeling" (1941).[161] From the USA where it originated, the sect first established itself in Burgas, Bulgaria in 1901. His observations were carried out together with Dr. Sharankov in 1934 through a classical anthropological field study, taking place during a fair in Turski Trustenik, a village in the Nikopol region of Northern Bulgaria, and the study included stenographic records of what had been literally shared with them.

Glossolalia means talking in unintelligible, non-existent languages, and is most commonly expressed through a verbal "salad" of chaotic syllable

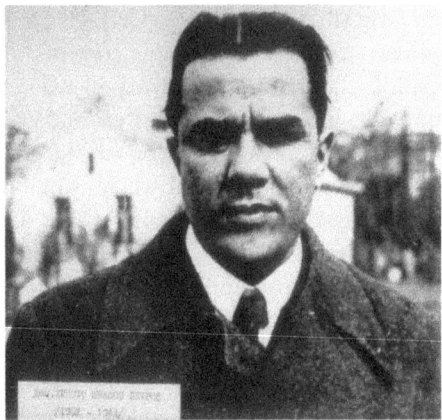

Fig. 8: Hristo Petrov (1901–1944)

combinations, while xenoglossia is the spontaneous ability to speak foreign and known languages. Members of the sect regard their skills as "extraordinary gifts" given to them by the Apostles and, hence, as signs of their connection to the Holy Spirit. Their faith drives them to consciously aspire to this "gift" and to maintain it when gained. Those that have gained it are considered privileged and in special connection to God, and are even believed to be able to merge with Him when falling into peculiar states.

The content of these beliefs materializes and directly reflects in psychopathology. The sect's ideology encourages dependent behaviors with its dogma that evil is solely the work of the Devil, rather than that of people, and so personal responsibility is taken away. Rejection of personal responsibility and even of one's own personality, in the author's apt expression, "clears the terrain for the Holy Spirit's invasion".[161] That is why children who can easily change their identity and speech have no particular difficulty in acquiring this "gift", as well. Eight cases of children with glossolalia, all with signs of marked physical and psychological developmental problems, and several cases in adults, among them one with epilepsy, are described. The course of the fits was identical: prodromes with tension, ecstasy, convulsions, and consequent indiscriminate, often contagious, and inarticulate yelling. The state approximated mental automatism syndrome with Séglas' psychomotor verbal hallucinations, albeit excluding the possibility of imitation, ostentation, or fraud. Pronounced psychic infantilism, suggestibility, aptitude for imitation, and contagious behaviors were observed in all of the interviewed participants, along with overt simulation in some of them. That is why the main interpretation of the mechanism behind this phenomenon is the compensation for personal failures. The personal neglect and impoverishment of all participants once they joined the sect are pointed out as evidence for the dysfunctional character of Pentecostals—as opposed to the adaptability of genuine religiosity.[161] At that time, some members faced lawsuits because of their refusal to perform regular military service. To qualify the phenomenon as an antipode of genuine religiosity, the author cites Paul the Apostle: "Wherefore tongues are for a sign, not to them that believe, but to them that believe not" (Corinthians I: 14–22).

Several decades later, I had the opportunity to observe some cases of glossolalia in female patients with schizophrenia and schizoaffective disorder who had briefly attended Pentecostal gatherings in the past. Suggestibility and imitation in these cases cannot serve as a convincing explanation for undeniable first-rank symptoms. Nevertheless, a certain dissociative nuance could be perceived in their psychotic experiences, with an ecstatic touch along with narrowed consciousness and, sometimes, ostentatious mannerisms—but these were present only during the glossolalia recital, not alongside the other symptoms. A patient with over 40 years of service in the sect showed a tendency to rhyme ("pok–tok–ok–ot–frock coat…"), which was missing in her speech outside of the glossolalia fits. It is likely that with the decline of the sect's popularity, it is increasingly becoming a retreat for patients facing serious mental illnesses in comparison with its earlier years.

In 1945 and 1946 Prof. Sharankov (Fig. 9) made his first descriptions of fire dancing, usually with icons, during the feast days of Saints Konstantin and Elena at the end of May or the beginning of June in the villages of Bulgari, near Tzarevo, and Novo Panicharevo, near Primorsko, both in the Burgas region of South-Eastern Bulgaria, and continued to follow up with them for decades. The described cases contain detailed biographical records and first-person narratives about the experience, particularly regarding the unusual states before entering the fire. This state is most frequently called capture, invasion, or conversion, while one of the interviewees, granny Kera from the village of Bulgari, calls it "swooning" and granny Zlata from the same village calls it "torment" ("… I have not been tormented lately"). The achievement of conversion, and subsequently being "captured, lost in reverie", is a sign of possession and affiliation to the society of *nestinari* or fire dancers. It is reached via self-absorption, frequently combined with refusing to eat or drink water. The other inhabitants can discern the "caught" or "tormented" one, and so avoid and leave her or him alone. As with Pentecostals, the state is consciously sought after and, as a result, predisposed personalities achieve peculiar voluntary depersonalization. Descriptions

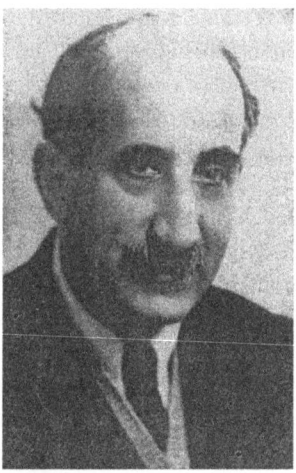

Fig. 9: Emanuil Sharankov (1903–1997)

of their "reverie" reveal a convincing dissociative narrowing of consciousness with scanty visual and auditory hallucinations during the episodes (but not outside of them), as well as conversion anesthesia and partial loss of memory afterwards. The author draws a parallel between fire dancing and hysteria. There is only one certain case of another pathology: an epileptic woman from the village of Bulgari.

As in a real cultural anthropological journey, the individual stories are examined in their geographic, social, and religious contexts, including such details as income, livelihood, and crime rates in the region.[186] The cult of fire can be traced back to the ancient cult of Mitra in Persia, and was transferred during the Roman Empire to the Balkans, where it took root in the Strandzha mountains of Southeastern Bulgaria. The author defines the *nestinari* (Fig. 10) as an independent religious community, the product of a special welding of pagan and Christian ritualism: "… a religious play associated with fire and accompanied by peculiar religious reverie".[186] Besides Mitraism, analogues have been made with the epidemics of demon possession in Medieval convents ("Here we go… and this one will also shout"), the "recklessly dancing", "stigmatized", and "convulsing" ones; *klikushestvo* in Russia (from the Russian *klikush*, to shout, meaning states with fits of yelling, barking, crowing, hitting oneself, and convulsions); and Pentecostals with their states of religious exultation. During his follow up of the custom over several decades after the first description, Sharankov attempted to

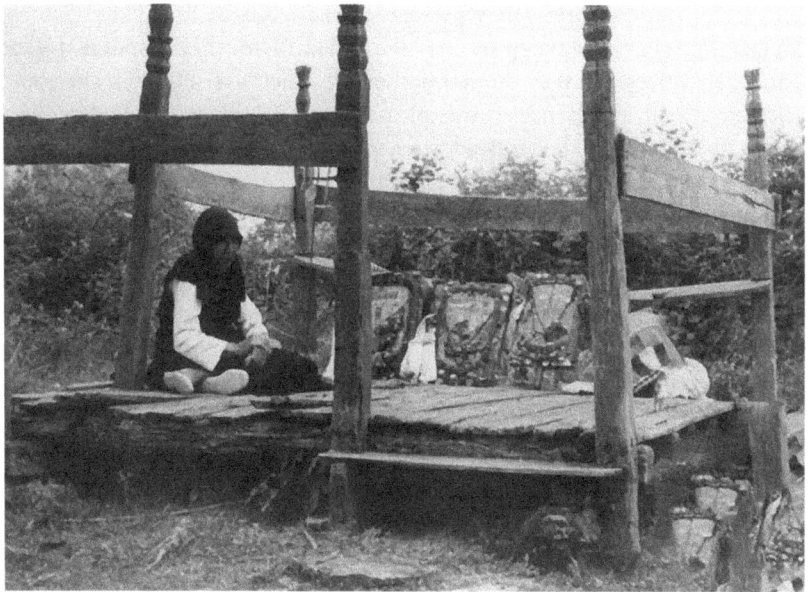

Fig. 10: Granny Zlata from the village of Bulgari, the last genuine nestinar in the Strandzha mountains

outline the personality profile of *nestinari* by means of questionnaires, also indicating the decline of the practice and its degradation into a tourist attraction.

The observed "extra sense" psychoses of the early 90s are a contemporary version of possession states. After decades of dogmatic atheism under communism, the new social environment saw superstitions, clairvoyance, magic, miraculous cures, and pseudo-scientific insights and kitsch blended with Orthodox rites gaining new ground. Some dramatic clinical pictures have also been observed, predominantly in women—possession by aliens and automatically writing under their dictation, and the abilities to tell fortunes and find cures, as well as sticking forks and spoons to the breasts, among other "extra-sensory" phenomena.

Clinical case. An 18-year-old girl, beaten and abused by her alcoholic father, experienced bouts of fainting with "deafness" four times but was still aware of what was happening around her. After an EEG and consultations with different specialists, a diagnosis of epilepsy was excluded. She visited a psychic who summoned spirits and had visions from the girl's future. After the visit, the patient became sad and detached and started communicating with extra-terrestrial creatures—they presented themselves as Rocky and Saturn. Contact was always initiated by her: she called them, they responded—she heard their voices, but they did not bother her otherwise, although she could feel their invisible presence. It was pleasant and soothing, and their voices, though heard only inside her head, were soft and deep-toned. She asked them questions about everyday life (e.g., whether her father would get drunk or whether her friend's boyfriend would leave her) and received specific answers. Sometimes, when they were "banned" from speaking, but not from communicating in other ways, she asked her questions in writing and received written replies through her hand being moved by an invisible force. Twice in a state of relaxation and "deafness" she had visions, one of which involved her being transformed into a goat; two male bears started chasing her before the vision disappeared.

Although she was admitted to the clinic with a diagnosis of acute psychosis, she was not given neuroleptic treatment. Her behavior was calm and conforming, and she shared her experiences with other patients and staff willingly, even with some boasting. She tried when asked to summon Rocky and Saturn, but announced that they would not appear in everybody's presence. She was discharged soon after without psychotic symptoms and without prescribed therapy. 24 years later, she is married, with two children from two marriages. She is extraverted, with a vivid but balanced temperament, has a job, is well adapted, and has had no relapses of psychosis, fits, or other abnormal behaviors.

Despite being brief and induced, the described state is nevertheless psychotic and dissociative in essence. The favorable characteristics are obvious: comprehensibility in the family context, specific provocation, quick recovery, the impression of playfulness and coquetting with her symptoms, and the lack of a dysfunctional impact on her behavior. The theme of communication with extraterrestrials is banal, trivial, and as if drawn from a schoolgirl's lexicon. Her lack of relapse years after the episode confirms the appropriateness of the clinical decision not to prescribe antipsychotics. This decision was made easier by the observation of the patient's attitude toward the symptoms: instead of controlling her behavior, as in the case of genuine psychosis, the patient controlled the "hallucinations", bringing them to life whenever she decided, thereby deriving a secondary gain from their prestigious status in the boulevard subculture, while at the same time preserving connection with reality and accessibility for feedback. This is not to imply her conscious imitation or simulation of psychosis. The mechanism is dissociative and includes a peculiar aspect in the genesis of reactive psychosis—the possibility of it being caused by experiences at one's *will*, not just by traumatic ones.

Clinical case. A 24-year-old female artist with interests in occult practices, paranormal literature, and clairvoyance, started hearing the voice of a famous psychic fortune-teller and began perceiving in her own thoughts, as if suggested by the fortune-teller, that she would hurt her father and her sister. She felt profound fear that she might be made to do evil against her will until she began to hear the voice of a more powerful "magus" ("the wise man from Sofia") who consoled and admonished her, neutralizing the psychic's suggestions. She felt his energy over her body erotically, as well as his thoughts in her head. She was treated in the clinic and discharged with improvement.

Despite maintenance neuroleptic treatment, after six months she claimed that she was the daughter of aliens, that the aliens wanted to destroy our world, and that she could predict the future. She was excited, violent, and either hostile or in a state of ecstasy. She claimed that the aliens Kiko (good) and Kino (evil) were fighting over her and that, depending on who prevailed and penetrated into her, the lamps would emit light in different ways and the weather would change. After the second hospitalization and a longer period of treatment, she partially recovered, yet remained more withdrawn and timid, spending more time in a village where she felt more relaxed. A year later, her relatives noticed that she had started to seclude herself and call on spirits in secret so that she wouldn't be "locked up in a mental hospital". She thought that the village grannies envied her abilities to call on spirits and rule over the "penetrations", and, for some time, it seemed to her that her spirit had possessed her dog—and vice versa. She started practicing contra-magic to fight against and eliminate the existing magical and alien thoughts ("… rushing suddenly, from above or through the mouth, possessing my inner space …"). During another hospitalization, improvement was achieved only after the application of thioproperazine in high doses. Since then, despite brief psychotic exacerbations and a moderate preoccupation with magic, her state has been stabilized; she has a job and is on maintenance treatment with a depot-neuroleptic.

As compared to the previous case, possession by spirits and aliens here constitutes the content of severe psychosis exhibiting gross loss of contact with reality and self-control, deterioration of behavior and functioning, relapses, and a chronic course. First-rank symptoms in this case do not play out as dissociative, and the interest in the paranormal is not a harmless hobby. The first episodes had the pattern of acute psychoses with an intense affect fluctuating between fear and ecstasy, without prominent polymorphism, however, but rather with the steady thread of a delusional plot tightly connected to external influences, no matter their origin (fortune-tellers, spirits, aliens, the village grannies). The specific nuances of her bodily and mental boundaries being grossly violated, along with the course of the disorder and the mild interpolated negative symptoms, make the diagnosis of schizophrenia unquestionable. In both of the presented cases, intense self-suggestibility precedes psychosis, though the ensuing clinical manifestations featured totally different courses. As with the cases from Pemba, the syndrome of possession is clinically heterogeneous and belongs to different states. The syndrome's context and impact on functioning, not the narrative for the possession itself, are crucial to the diagnosis and treatment approach.

8 Schizophrenia and Culture

> There is only one difference between a madman and me.
> The madman thinks he is sane. I know I am mad.
>
> S. Dali

If schizophrenia did not exist, it probably could have been invented. It is undoubtedly the most interesting and enigmatic human pathology that continues to puzzle and fascinate with the richness and incomprehensibility of its clinical manifestations. The connection between this illness and culture is fundamental to the debate between universalists and relativists in transcultural psychiatry. The WHO's worldwide comparative studies of schizophrenia convincingly show its universality as a mental disorder, with similar prevalence and manifestation in different populations.[88, 98] Nevertheless, some essential differences can be outlined according to cultural contexts: in the disease's epidemiology, manifestation, course, and outcome.

These differences are not easy to explain through the paradigm of universal genetic illnesses. Genetic contribution to schizophrenia may reach 50 %—with the highest degree of concordance in monozygotic twins, indicating that at least half of the reasons lie outside of the genotype, e.g., viruses or ecological, social, or other factors. Contemporary genetic studies on copy number variations (CNVs) and single nucleotide polymorphisms (SNPs) reveal the role of de novo mutations with approximately similar rates in each generation.[171] This role in turn has a phenomenological projection. Around 80 % of all patients with schizophrenia are sporadic cases, i.e., with no relatives experiencing overt pathologies, in contrast to the affective disorders which have higher occurrences in family histories. More severe clinical pictures (such as regressive hebephrenic states) tend to be even more sporadic, while the least severe cases (e.g., schizoaffective forms) tend to more often be associated with a family history.

Since people with schizophrenia rarely have children, natural selection should lead to the disappearance of the illness. Its sustainability through generations, however, suggests that the de novo mutations compensating for lack of offspring could likely be associated with some *evolutionary advantage*. These mutations increase the risk of pathology in a broad spectrum—from schizophrenia and autism to syndromes with physical aberrations and mental retardation. It might be hypothesized whether or not the onset of schizophrenia protects against more severe pathologies.

At the same time, this sustainability across generations is uncertain and has been observed only for approximately the last century. Historical descriptions of states resembling schizophrenia are surprisingly absent from ancient texts. This cannot be attributed to a lack of keen observation; on the contrary, the clinical descriptions of ancient healers such as Hippocrates, Aretaeus of Cappadocia, and Avicenna (e.g., of mania and depression) are amazingly trustworthy and vivid. The Prophet Ezekiel and King Nebuchadnezzar in the Old Testament are described as having experienced psychotic states, but also with such organic and regressive signs as coprophagia, lycanthropy, and brutalization. The first inpatient facilities for the mentally ill in the Middle Ages—whether in Baghdad, Cairo, Valencia, Zaragoza, Toledo, Uppsala, Elbing, or London—were crowded with people suffering from infectious organic states, dementia, and physical diseases, as well as vagrants seeking shelter because meals were served three times a day there and wine was also poured out for therapeutic purposes. Descriptions bearing a convincing resemblance to schizophrenia appeared only later, e.g., the Fool in Shakespeare's King Lear. It turns out that clinical manifestations either underwent major changes over time or that schizophrenia was truly a *new* disease, present only since the 17th century.[96] According to some authors, there was a real increase of schizophrenia cases in Western Europe and North America following the end of the 18th century, coinciding with the mass introduction of the smallpox vaccine (hence, the hypothesis for modification of the variola virus as one possible etiology). The growing prevalence was already well documented by the 19th century, but this actually reflects better recognition for the sake of isolation and treatment in the period of expansion for psychiatry practiced in asylum-type hospitals. In the 1960s, a comparative study in the UK and USA[41]—a pilot one for the subsequent WHO global initiatives—found differences in the countries' respective diagnostic practices: while the over-diagnosis of schizophrenia was widespread in the US, at the same time the disease was diagnosed much more conservatively in the UK. This finding confirmed that differences in prevalence rates may simply be an artifact of the diagnostic process.

There are other hypotheses and indirect evidence which support schizophrenia as a relatively *new illness* in human history, though it has existed for more than a few centuries. Its origin can be provisionally referred to as the first appearance of differentiated speech approximately 10,000–12,000 years ago.[210] Its frequency in the course of human history is unknown. Probably after its initial appearance some 500 or 600 human generations ago, it remained relatively rare, with an increase in prevalence rates over the last few centuries and a trend towards gradual decrease during the last several decades.[100] Some mental disorders have analogues in animals and pre-historic humans, but such an analogue is missing for schizophrenia. It is a genuinely human disease. In a phylogenetic context, the mystery of its origin attains specific meaning. There is some evidence that along with underdeveloped speech and a tendency to externalize "inner" speech, hearing voices was normal for the human race more than 12,000 years ago. The same applies to sensing the presence of aliens and outer influences on archaic self-structures where the boundary between one's inner and outer (collective) world was uncertain. These experiences transmuted themselves into pathology only after the differentiation of homo sapiens as individual beings, apart from the horde's collective self. In the course of this development, the mechanism for differentiation between one's own thoughts from one's own words and from others' words, as well as their semantic decoding, can be affected.[44] Despite clinical variability, the core syndrome in schizophrenia bears the signs of such confusion on the level of speech and semantics. Thereby, the appearance of schizophrenia combined with differentiated speech in human phylogenesis offers good reason to view it as the evolutionary price that mankind has paid for the development of speech.[44, 210] Presumably, schizophrenia is a product of the complex epigenetic interplay between mutations and their filtering by way of cultural evolution.

8.1 Epidemiology

The cliché that schizophrenia affects around one percent of the global population is usually followed by a false impression that this rate is universal, masking the facts that average prevalence rates are generally lower and that variations across different populations exist in a *very broad scope*. The prevalence rate (the number of cases per 1,000 individuals in the general population) varies between 2.7 and 8.3 per 1,000,[141] with the median lifetime prevalence rate being 4.0 per 1,000 and the median of lifetime morbidity risk at 7.2 per 1,000. Point prevalence (the number of symptomatic cases at a given moment) is around 5 per 1,000. The incidence rate (the number of first-onset cases, usually for a single year, in the general population) averages 20 per 100,000 annually, but in fact varies between 11 and 70 per 100,000 on a yearly basis.[141, 208] The onset usually comes in adolescence, with its average peak in males occurring 9 years earlier than in females.[197,208] The lifetime morbidity risk for schizophrenia in men is 30–40 % higher than in women, and the ratio of men to women among affected individuals is 1.4: 1. The so-called class gradient, i.e., that a higher prevalence rate exists among people from lower social classes, those living in ghettos, and the marginalized, is nearly a regular finding. In Bulgaria, the prevalence rate is

3.84 per 1,000 according to statistics published by the state mental health services, a number which is very close to figures given in the dispensary registers some decades ago, and also to the findings from 1974 in the only survey in the country ever done about the epidemiology of schizophrenia with an outreach search in a geographically defined region (in Sofia).[96]

Prevalence and incidence depend on different factors. Apart from etiology, prevalence also depends strongly on demographic, social, and other environmental factors. For instance, the average life expectancy of people with schizophrenia is nearly 15 years lower than the average within respective local populations, and this has a direct influence on their percentage of the population. The number of first-onset cases is, however, relatively independent of these factors. For this reason, it should be expected for the indicator incidence to be closer to the underlying etiology than prevalence, and, hence, for it to be more stable and invariant in different cultures.

The incidence rates in eight of the centers participating in the International Pilot Study of Schizophrenia (IPSS) and the Determinants of Outcome of Severe Mental Disorders (DOSMED) study are 3.7 and 4.8 per 10,000 for men and women, respectively, when applying a "broad" definition of schizophrenia.[88] The lowest rate for men (1.8) is found in Aarhus, Denmark, and in Honolulu, Hawaii, with the lowest for women (1.2) also being found in Aarhus. The difference between the rates across centers is statistically significant. When applying a "narrow" definition of schizophrenia (the CATEGO class S+ criteria, corresponding in general to Schneider's first-rank symptoms), both the results and their variations are lower—from 0.8 in Aarhus to 1.4 in Nottingham, England, for both men and women. The lowest rate for men (0.8) is found in the urban region of Chandigarh, India, and the highest one (1.7) is in Nottingham, England—while the lowest rate for women (0.5) is again found in Aarhus. The highest for women (1.4) is in Moscow, Russia. The differences between rates across centers when the "narrow" definition is used are not statistically significant among men, yet they are at the threshold of statistical significance among women, i.e., the actual frequencies of first-onset cases are more similar across centers when restricting the definition of the illness. This supports the idea that the "central" syndrome in schizophrenia emerges with almost equal probability within different populations.[88] Summarizing all reliable studies, however, the range of data variations expands— from 11 to 70 per 100,000, thus exceeding the range of variations in prevalence rates.[141] Such a confusing tendency in the frequency of schizophrenia onset is only compatible with the presence of intrinsic differences between cultures.

Findings of lower or higher than average frequencies in some populations are intriguing. Lower rates have been detected at different times and with different methods in Thuringia and Bavaria in Germany, and Uzbekistan in the former USSR, as well as among the native population of Taiwan before Chinese settlement and in the northern part of Papua New Guinea. In the latter, isolated from the rest of the island by a high mountain range and lacking practically any population exchanges, the incidence is 0.03 per 1,000 and the prevalence is only 0.19 per 1000, rates which are several times lower than those found on the rest of the island.[147] It is claimed that there are no human subpopulations without any recognized cases of schizophrenia, although this may not hold true for some traditional communities in the Amazon River basin or among the Maasai in East Africa. The absence or extreme rarity of schizophrenia in these communities confirms that it may be a relatively new illness. The languages and mentalizations of these tribes are not very developed, and that is why schizophrenia—the peculiar historical artifact of language development and the process of mentalization—is very rare or probably absent. On the other hand, it is possible that, due to huge cultural differences with other human populations, schizophrenia may have other clinical manifestation in these tribes and thus remains unrecognized.

Higher frequencies of schizophrenia have been found in the following: a region in Northern Sweden with a morbidity risk of 2.68 % for women and 2.27 % for men and with a prevalence rate 3 times above the country average; Ireland, where the prevalence rate is four times higher than in England;[88] the Istrian peninsula on the Adriatic Sea, with a prevalence rate exceeding 40 % of the average for Croatia; the southeastern part of Canada's Baffin Island; and among the Tamil people in India.[100] Most of these regions constitute isolates with favorable conditions for genetic segregation, increasing the effect of the illness of some predecessor on their offspring, as well as for high concentrations of infectious diseases, particularly rubella and measles—which may have some relation to the etiology of schizophrenia. Cultural differences are noticeable through the distinctions between similar populations with a common ethnic background and a common physical environment, such as Norway and Iceland: there is a higher rate of schizophrenia in Norway than there is in Iceland. The highest rate of the illness among the three major ethno-religious groups on Mauritius is in Africans, followed by Indian Hindus, with the lowest rate occurring in Indian Muslims.[20] Rates a couple of times higher than average have been estimated in the central, most densely populated parts of large metropolitan areas and among immigrants, particularly from the Caribbean, in some Western countries (this has been especially well documented in the UK and the Netherlands), with rates still remaining high among second-generation immigrants.[105, 141, 147]

Some plausible explanations for differences in the spread of schizophrenia come down to certain distinctions in expressed emotions in different cultures. These distinctions affect clinical manifestations of the disease in the domains of emotion and volition as well as the threshold of recognition by others. Other explanations refer to racial prejudices towards behaviors that appear to be different and inapprehensible. Whether or not cross-cultural studies comparing rates of schizophrenia in different populations do assess the same matter across different cultures remains an open question. Part of the answer will come from examining what we know about the clinical picture and the course of the illness.

8.2 Clinical Picture

The "central" schizophrenic syndrome, generally including first-rank symptoms (thought insertion, broadcasting and echo, commenting verbal hallucinations, delusions of control and submission to outer forces), is present in all cultures with approximately the same frequency. The ten most frequent symptoms of schizophrenia in the WHO studies overlap to a considerable degree with Schneider's syndrome, and are found in all cultures. They bear strong resemblances to magic rituals in some cultures with shamanic traditions. Within these cultures, however, such unusual states and talking with spirits—as part of the behavioral rite of the magus or healer—are clearly distinguished from what are considered to be signs of mental illness[135, 145, 172] (Chapter 6). Cultural differences concern nuances in the clinical manifestation, ratio between clinical forms, tolerance of morbid behaviors, course, and outcome of the illness.

The division of schizophrenia into separate clinical forms, despite its survival for over 100 years under the overwhelming authority of Kraepelin, is extremely provisory. The main reason for this is the absence of the forms' long-term stability. A patient with catatonic onset, for instance, may display paranoid-hallucinatory syndromes and may finish as in a hebephrenic outcome state. In the DSM-5, as expected, the forms have been eliminated. There exist more grounds for dividing the illness into distinct forms according to its course or the presence of negative symptoms, as well as other deficits or physical dysplasias, than there are according to the clinical picture. If, regardless, the division is based on clinical descriptions, then the replacement of the four classical forms—paranoid, catatonic, simple, and hebephrenic (or disorganized)—with a simpler division along the paranoid–non-paranoid line would be more stable and useful. This division roughly coincides with the one between non-deficit and deficit forms, and also has an association with endophenotype markers; therefore, it may successfully work towards the aims of researching an underlying etiology.

Categorization, however, does not reflect the richness of clinical manifestation. Any symptom or syndrome found in general psychopathology—from conversion to dementia—can exist in schizophrenia. At the same time, schizophrenia contains phenomena that are not encountered elsewhere. This diversity turns dementia praecox (a term borrowed by Kraepelin from the Czech neurologist A. Pick) into a genuine heir of the unitary psychosis (*Einheitspsychose*) of the 19th century, in contrast to Kraepelin's systematic dichotomy. It is impossible to embrace schizophrenia, let alone understand it, by ticking diagnostic criteria off a checklist. Beyond formal criteria, invisible threads weave the symptoms together into a general picture like a fine cobweb. The ghostly tangle of these threads is inhabited by: the discrete eccentricities of motorics and facial expression, a mixture of semantic layers inundated with both literal and figurative meaning, concreteness and abstraction, metaphor and prototype, and a fluidity of borders both between the physical and the mental and between inner and outer physical–mental realities; the materialization of mental phenomena (for instance, thoughts "weighing like stones"); and the mentalization of physical objects, idiosyncrasies concerning conventional meanings, self-sufficiency, detaching from one's own perceptions, and attributing alien characteristics to one's own physiological and psychological processes. The gradual seclusion from the material world and sinking into solipsism without demands, aims, or boredom brings about a final stage where what is not happening has priority over what is happening, and both verbalization and conventional categorization turn, to borrow one patient's expression, into "trivialities".

The paranoid form is the most common of the classical clinical forms. It is more frequently present in developed countries, where positive syndromes are more prolific and richer, with more complicated plots and more frequent paraphrenias. In the Old World intellectual tradition, which can be most apparently recognized in the interpretations of Foucault,[58] complex delusional content transforms itself into a cultural metaphor: madness is woven into the very fabric of civilization. By contrast, in collectivistic cultures delusional stories lack salient systematization. There, psychotic behaviors often seem to be incomprehensible, without any motive or guiding delusional logic. Psychotic exacerbations are commonly manifest in the acute psychotic syndromes of the oneiroid or bouffée délirante type: with extreme delusional affect, disorganization, unpredictability, frequently recklessly destructive motorics, and scarce delusional productivity. In these, essentially cycloid (predominantly the motility type), sudden onset psychoses, there is usually a narrowing of consciousness which thus resembles either delirium or an acute dissociative reaction. A differential diagnosis is imperative because delirium caused by infectious diseases and acute dissociative confusion states are both common in the Third World. On the other hand, the cerebral form of trypanosomiasis may present symptoms similar to "insidious onset", imitating "European" schizophrenia onset.

Other differences in phenomenology include a higher frequency of visual hallucinations in Africa, along with a marked tolerance towards hearing voices to the extent that they are perceived as non-pathological signs. In Nigeria, for instance, among the Yoruba people in rural regions commonly display acute confusional states with emotional lability and retrospective ecmnesias associated with past hallucinatory experiences, while in urban regions clinical conditions similar to "Western" ones prevail.[100] In Hawaii, autistic traits are more common among people of Japanese descent, while acute agitated states are more common among Filipinos and Polynesians.

There are also distinctions concerning some aspects of the delusional story: for example, a patient's claim that he is growing his father's hair on his own skin should match up to a bizarre categorization, but in some traditional communities where one's connection to kin is strong and literal, such a claim would not be considered strange. A cultural comparison between two patients with the same delusional claims from Bulgaria and Tanzania shows a poorer prognosis for the former patient (the bizarreness itself complicated the prognosis) as compared to the latter, whose story was not unusual for the cultural context. The same rule also applied in this case to parallel realities as a delusional topic. A patient with from an African subculture who shared identical delusional subject matter did not meet the criteria for paraphrenia because of the absence of the delusions' systematization (intrinsic to the story of the European paraphrenic patient), despite their fantastic characteristics and expansiveness. Because of this, the Tanzanian patient's illness course and individual prognosis were different from the Bulgarian analogue, despite the literal sameness of subject matter in both patients' delusions.

In reciprocity to the paranoid form, catatonic and hebephrenic conditions are rarer in developed countries than they are in the Third World. Relevant cultural differences here, however, are the result of environmental physical factors. It seems that geographical borders in reference to the distribution of infectious diseases overlap to a high degree with borders distinguishing ratios between the clinical forms. These differences are clearly exhibited in catatonia. Described for the first time by Kahlbaum in his small and notable 1874 monograph *Catatonia or Tension Insanity*,[110] it still remains a puzzle today. Kahlbaum viewed the syndrome as a stage in the display of unitary psychosis, a very influential diagnostic construct at that time. If the criteria of modern classifications were applied to the 25 clinical descriptions from his monograph, most of them would be diagnosed today with organic or affective disorders—but not as schizophrenia. Under the authority of Kraepelin, however, catatonia was considered a form of schizophrenia for almost a century after he attached it to dementia praecox in the fourth edition of his textbook. This was also in spite of unvarying stipulations made by Leonhard and many other proficient clinicians about its more specific status. Clinical practice shows that catatonia is most frequently not an independent syndrome or clinical form, but rather a stage in the development of psychotic episodes—similar not only to Kahlbaum's interpretation from the 19th century, but also to current views on the psychotic continuum as opposed to Kraepelin's traditional dichotomy.[42] Further observations additionally suggest that catatonia may be a phenocopy of non-mental pathologies.

The organic origin of most catatonias has been validated by trends in their distribution over the course of time. All the empirical data point out that they have shown historic tendency to decrease in developed countries, especially during the second half of the 20th century. In the USA, they accounted for 6-15 % of all adult patients hospitalized in mental health facilities;[36] in England, this percentage decreased from 6 % to 0.5 % between 1850 and 1950; and the same trend occurred in Finland, where from 1953 to 1993 it dropped from 37 % to 11 %.[55] In the WHO IPSS study,[221] clear distinctions were detected in the frequencies of the catatonic forms between national samples: on the one hand, Agra, India—15.7 %, Cali, Columbia—10.2 %, and Ibadan, Nigeria—6.9 %, and, on the other hand, Aarhus, Denmark—1.5 %, London—2.3 %, Moscow—0 %, Prague—0 %, Washington, D.C. —0.75 %, and Taipei, Taiwan—2.2 %. Frequency was steadily high in all centers from the Third World, where infectious diseases prevail as the dominant portion of global illness, and was low in developed countries.

A common cause of catatonic syndromes, as well as of other phenocopies of functional psychoses, is cerebral malaria. Most catatonic cases attributed to schizophrenia are, in fact, due to organic, prevailingly infectious causes. Their decrease in developed countries ran historically in parallel to the eradication of infectious diseases—and this deduction is in accord with the retrospective diagnosis of Kahlbaum's clinical cases. The variable origin of catatonia in modern classifications[6, 222] has been confirmed particularly conclusively in the DSM, which in its fourth edition also included organic catatonic syndrome ("due to a general medical condition") and a separate descriptor for catatonic features in affective and other disorders.

The downturn of catatonia (Fig. 11) in developed countries has brought about a practical non-recognition of its clinical manifestations. Overt symptoms such as waxy flexibility, stupor, echo phenomena, posing, or reckless agitation are inserted in the diagnostic criteria, however, they frequently go even unrecognized

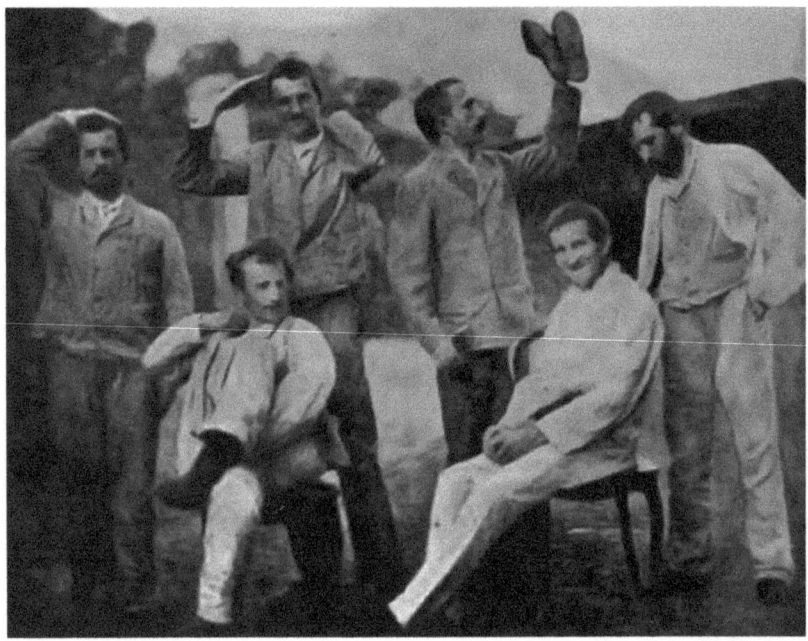

Fig. 11: Patients with catatonia, illustration from Kraepelin's textbook, 1899 edition

and are not distinguished from other organic states. Apart from these, other less common and more discrete symptoms include: opposition or mirror movements, ambitendency, *gegenhalten* (increasing resistance to attempts to change one's posture), a grasping reflex, *mitgehen* (movement by inertia in one direction after a minimal push with a finger, despite instructions to halt); automatic obedience (even to dangerous tasks), stereotypical wrinkling, coughing, knocking, slapping, snoring, clicking of the tongue, or snorting; and formal, dry and stiff speech (including the *vouvoyer* phenomenon among French speakers, i.e., addressing close relatives with the polite plural form). The essence of the syndrome is one's motor behavior being detached from inner experiences—much like in dissociative phenomena and regress.

Febrile catatonia is a rare and frequently fatal condition, also described as lethal or malignant catatonia,[55, 195] which, in essence, is severe encephalopathy. Its key features are stupor with confusion, hyperthermia, muscle rigidity (with or without catalepsy), hypo or hypertension, tachycardia, sweating, incontinence, and the absence of consistent paraclinical findings. Specific catatonic signs are in fact very few in number. As with catatonia in general, febrile catatonia is a syndrome, not a diagnosis. The more severe the condition, the less evident are the catatonic signs—at the expense of the general brain toxic symptoms, which prevail in the clinical picture and determine the outcome. The condition can be a peak escalation of syndromes on a trajectory of the psychotic continuum, similar to the antiquated unitary psychosis, and indicative of the limitations of categorical diagnoses. Severe general brain symptoms require their distinction apart from physical diseases with amentia. The cultural differences in these severe organic conditions rest on the predominance of amentia, due to cerebral forms of infectious diseases in the Third World.

Much closer to the core defects of schizophrenia are its negative symptoms—what Kraepelin labeled the "atrophy of emotions" and "perversion of volition". For this reason, their distribution should be more adherent to universal tendencies rather than cultural specifics. Negative symptoms are indeed present in all cultures, but in some of them a professional "outsider" to the culture may have difficulty in identifying them. They may be hardly distinguished from states of gloomy seclusion for ritual reasons, signs of shame or being rejected by the community, or from an ascetic, hermit's life. The negative symptoms—avolition, alogia, anhedonia, apathy, affective flattening, disturbed attention, and inappropriate affect[7]—represent the decrease or loss of experiences or behaviors that are normally present in individuals from the *same* culture. They include deficits in subjective experience, such as a decreased desire for intimacy, lower motivation, and the inability to feel pleasure, as well as in one's outward expression, e.g., of emotions and speech. The manifestations in different spheres require assessment through different sources: self-assessment, clinical judgment, and data from staff and relatives.

The emphasis on a separate and precise assessment does not allow for genuine negative symptoms to be associated with their respective consequences. Some authors attach poor hygiene to the symptoms, but this is not a symptom, *per se*; it is rather their consequence. While symptoms are closer to the core defect and as such are more invariant and universal, the consequences are less distinguishing and have more cultural variations, yet personal neglect is universal.

Factor analyses of clinical manifestations, both of schizophrenia and its negative symptoms, demonstrate a certain universality of the syndrome's structure. In schizophrenia, as it has been analyzed in different studies, three factors are usually isolated: negative, positive, and disorganization.[126] Other studies have isolated five instead of three: negative, positive, agitation, depression, and cognitive, but this detracts from the much clearer and more consolidated three-factor model—depression can be assigned to the negative syndrome, while agitation and cognitive disturbance fall under the disorganization syndrome. As for the factor structure of the negative syndrome (in itself invariable within the factor structure of schizophrenia), two factors are usually isolated: motivation/pleasure and expression,[200] diminished expression and disordered relating,[53] or reduced expression and anhedonia-asociality,[24] according to the denominations in the rating scales for negative symptoms used in the studies.[8, 124] Factor analysis using SANS, probably the most reliable scale in this area, has further isolated other factors with lower eigenvalues, such as alogia and disturbance of attention.[24] They are products of a too-broad categorization (into five factors, rather than three) because along with the inappropriate affect, a zone of overlap is reflected between the negative and disorganization syndromes. The two-factor structure, particularly of diminished expression and disordered relating, has been reproduced in studies in other populations such as the South African Xhosa,[53] which demonstrates that the factor structure of schizophrenia's symptoms, and especially of its negative symptoms, is relatively independent of cultural differences.

8.3 Course and Outcome

Data from the 1970s onward have not supported Kraepelin's view of the invariable deterioration and poor outcome, yet it has persisted regardless. This view is so deeply embedded in psychiatrists' professional mentality that any new data have been met with mistrust. According to the classical research: around half of all patients display an undulating course with partial or full remissions followed by relapses; around one third have a chronic, continuous course with a poor prognosis; and only a small portion reach recovery and a good outcome. Results published in the 1970s—an intense follow-up by M. Bleuler[26] of 208 patients over 20 years which showed that more than half of them significantly improved after a long illness—caused genuine surprise. Analogous results were obtained by large follow-up studies in Italy,[39] the UK,[140] Germany,[89] and other European countries,[11] as well as in North America[80]—and the length of some of them lasted over 32 years.[80] One of the largest catamnestic samples in schizophrenia was carried out by the Bulgarian author A. Marinov, who continued his follow-up with 636 patients for decades: 58 % of them successfully completed the end point of assessment—36 % of them with full remission, and 54 % with chronic symptoms.[137]

These studies reflect the course of illness in only Europe and North America, and do not clarify whether this tendency is a global one or whether the characteristics of schizophrenia, including course and outcome, are similar everywhere. The answer to these questions lie in the large-scale WHO studies starting

Tab. 4: Results from the International Pilot Study of Schizophrenia (IPSS) in different cultures, follow up for 26 years

Center	Specifics	Outcome
Agra, India	Overpopulation, Hindi, Islam, family support, most patients without hospitalizations or maintenance treatment	73.8 % full remission, 48 % of men and 81 % of women well-functioning (GAF-D>81)
Cali, Columbia	Civil war, drug cartels, outpatient network, health promotion	1/2 without significant symptoms, 3/4 well-functioning, 2/3 employed
Prague, Czech Republic	Social transition, growing crime rate, developed hospital psychiatry	1/2 recovered, large portion in hospitals and nursing homes, and on neuroleptics

in the 1960s for testing hypotheses about the disease's universality. They include sample centers from different continents and social systems, and with differing degrees of industrial development which have been assessed with similar methods and identical instruments. There is a sizeable Bulgarian contribution to their planning and implementation.[67, 68, 100, 101] These studies are sometimes summarized as the International Study of Schizophrenia (ISoS),[88] yet they actually comprise three separate studies: The International Pilot Study of Schizophrenia (IPSS), Determinants of Outcomes and Course of Severe Mental Disorders (DOSMED), and Reduction and Assessment of Psychiatric Disability (RAPyD). In total, ISoS is carried out in 18 centers from 14 countries on every continent, with 1,740 patients being assessed over the course of 12 to 26 years. The method itself has come into criticism because of the forceful homogenizing of groups, with its possible overestimation of universality, and the neglect of cultural specifics.[119]

The main results across centers are concisely summarized in Tabs. 4, 5, and 6, juxtaposing specifics of the environment, sample, and health care with basic indicators of outcome—e.g., severity of psychopathology, degree of social dysfunction, disability, portion of those taking neuroleptics, and those living in institutions. Notable diagnostic stability is observed: with 88 % of patients preserving their diagnoses within the spectrum of schizophrenia disorders, and stability being higher for schizophrenia than it is for schizoaffective forms and onsets with undifferentiated acute psychoses. 35 % of all patients have a favorable course, spending less than 15 % of the follow-up period in psychosis and without serious disadaptation for the remainder of time under study, while the most severe course is observed in only 19 % of all surveyed patients.

Tab. 5: Results from the Determinants of Outcomes and Course of Severe Mental Disorders (DOSMED) in different cultures, follow up for 15 years

Center	Specifics	Outcome
Chandigarh, India	Family support, attribution of illness to external causes, low stigma, most patients without hospitalization or neuroleptic treatment	75 % of urban and 81 % of rural patients without significant symptoms, >65 % well-functioning in the community, no homelessness
Dublin, Ireland	High level of stigma and high rate of hospitalizations, transition to community care	Only 1/3 with recovery, high disability and unemployment rate, 3/4 on neuroleptics
Honolulu, Hawaii	Modern forms of care, family support, continuous course predominates	69 % in the community, but also frequent hospitalizations and placement in nursing homes
Moscow, Russia	Developed ambulatory network, high rate of insidious onset, strict dispensary follow up, overcontrol	57.6 % with improvement, low rates of disability, most patients are employed
Nagasaki, Japan	High level of stigma, collective traumatic experience, long hospital stays, high rate of insidious onset and hebephrenia	1/3 recovery, 1/2 poor functioning, 57 % chronic course
Nottingham, England	Community psychiatry with small day centers, small wards, programs in patients' homes, individualized approach	69 % remittance, 58 % on neuroleptics, 95 % in the community, 64 % well-functioning
Rochester, USA	Multi-ethnic and religious environment, deinstitutionalization, short hospital stays	Severe psychopathology (only 25.9 % with GAF-S>70), >1/2 with disability

The main conclusion is that more than 60 % of the surveyed patients have "recovered", i.e., continue to only experience insignificant residual symptoms (Fig. 12). Almost half of all patients had no psychotic episodes during the last two years, and between half and three quarters of them have held a job for the better part of the last two years. Between 39 % and 49 % are well-functioning, according to the ratings of the DAS scale; and between half and two thirds of them have either no disability or have a mild disability, according to the ratings of the GAF-D scale. One of the worst outcomes is in the Bulgarian center (Sofia), where the majority of patients experience a chronic course, severe psychopathology, poor functioning, and unemployment. Paternalistic control, stigma, severity of

Course and Outcome 119

Tab. 6: Results from the Reduction and Assessment of Psychiatric Disability (RAPyD) in different cultures, follow up over 14 to 16 years

Center	Specifics	Outcome
Groningen, Netherlands	Lack of family support, sectorial organizational principle, focus on human rights, community care	52 % poor functioning, 23 % in hospitals and nursing homes, and high suicide rate—despite this, 60 % evaluated as recovered
Manheim, Germany	Reform in mental health care, community care	3/4 with episodic course, 1/4 with chronic course, 1/2 poor functioning, only 30 % employed
Sofia, Bulgaria	Social transition, paternalism, high family burden, stigma, isolation, lack of modern out-patient forms of care	41.8 % with chronic course, 52.8 % with severe psychopathology, 36.7 % with severe disability, difficulty in finding jobs

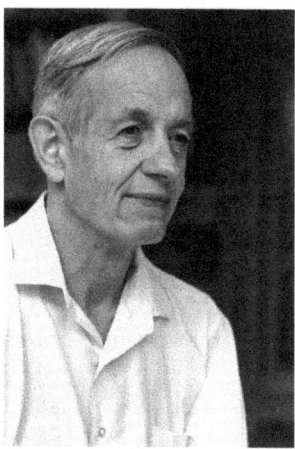

Fig. 12: John Nash, Nobel prize winner in economics, diagnosed with schizophrenia (Courtesy to Getty Images)

the burden of care on relatives, and family taboos are all exhibited.[67, 68] A considerable dissociation between the severity of psychopathology and social dysfunction is found in some centers, including the Bulgarian one: a lack of parallelism, and thence linear causality between the clinical picture and social impairment. Another lack of parallelism exists regarding the link between developed mental health care and poor outcomes, e.g., in some Western centers—as if to demonstrate that even sophisticated programs cannot compensate for alienation.

Patients with schizophrenia have more unfavorable characteristics, though not enough to be statistically significant, than those with non-schizophrenic psychoses. The majority of patients (between 70 and 85 %) live with their families and friends, while the inhabitants of chronic hospitals and nursing homes number between 4 and 15 %, and homelessness is a rarity. Only 8 % of patients have committed aggressive acts, most of them mild and not dangerous, 5 % have attempted suicide at least once, and comorbidity with alcohol or other psychoactive substances addiction is low. Lethality among patients with schizophrenia is higher than in the general population. In all three WHO studies, the outcome is consistently better in developing countries than it is in developed ones. The rate of recovery in Agra (India) in particular is one and a half times higher than the average for all other centers.

Even about one fifth of patients with poor prognostic factors at the onset and a poor course of illness early on (in the first 2 years) do reach late recovery. Chances for late recovery among this group is higher in developing countries (42 %) than in developed countries (33 %). The probability that patients with schizophrenia will get married in the Indian cohort is an average of 73 % (71 % for men and 74 % for women), while in the samples from developed countries, the average probability of marriage only reaches 38 % (28 % for men and 48 % for women). This finding depends on cultural pressures to create a family, as well as the status of parenthood within the community. In India, childbearing is a duty (*dharma*) which even mobilizes patients with schizophrenia to action: schizophrenia seems, to them, to be a lesser stigma than having no children. Negative symptoms are detected in less than half of patients faced with long-term illness. In half of all cases, the episodic course is more favorable regardless of either an acute or insidious onset.

The data show that late recovery in schizophrenia is realistic for at least half of all patients who are diagnosed, and that it is more common in the developing world than it is in developed countries. Recovery has a complex and non-homogeneous nature, while course and outcome depend on numerous factors. The most decisive role is played by the early period of the illness, particularly the amount of time in which the patient has been psychotic during the first two years—the lesser the amount, the more favorable the total course of the illness, the milder the disability and the more benevolent the symptom profile will be.[88] Predictors of poor outcome include negative symptoms, especially their insidious onset, a lack of family ties, loneliness, unemployment, a high premorbid social status, treatment resistance, cognitive disturbances, the abuse of alcohol or other psychoactive substances, and unfavorable personality traits.[88] Poorer prognoses in more developed countries are associated with competitive relationships, stigma, and a smaller number of family members sharing the care for their ill relative.

On the one hand, the expectations of patients, their families, and their doctors form a powerful recovery factor. Family connections and low levels of expressed emotions in traditional cultures have a mediating role in the disease's course and outcome. The responsibility of child rearing, for instance (with the aid of others, rather than as a single mother like in developed countries), can motivate psychotic patients to gain better control over their symptoms and treatment. The role of social factors—figuratively reflecting a broader family—is similar to that of real families: *tolerance* being the key to recovery in both of them. What it provides are reduced requirements for support and lower levels of stigma, discrimination, and social pressure.

9 Affective Disorder, Anxiety, and Culture

> Fear materializes what arouses it.
>
> *I. Bergman*

Emotions are universal and add meaning to life and events. Unlike the complex experiences of schizophrenia, they are archetypal, connected with human drives, and universally recognizable. People from different cultures can usually easily detect only through facial expressions the six basic emotions—anger, disgust, fear, happiness, sadness, and surprise (and a seventh, contempt, which is added by some authors). According to Darwin, emotional expression is universal not only for humans but also for gorillas.[46] Certain cultural differences exist in the acceptability, rules, and thresholds for expressing emotions. Individualistic cultures more often encourage the expression of negative emotions, while collectivistic ones encourage the positive, yet negative feelings are often expressed towards representatives of other groups.

The perception and decoding of emotions are also distinct. For instance, in many places in Africa smiling disguises anxiety, or other negative feelings which might be considered inappropriate for the situation by someone not familiar with the culture. There are also differences in the reasons, language, and meaning attributed to emotions. The words for many feelings cannot be precisely translated. In large linguistic families of the Third World, only one word is used to indicate both anger and sadness.[142, 181] The European localization of feelings in folklore is usually in the heart, while in Japan it is in the guts. The importance assigned to emotions (and to the psychotherapies which focus on them) in North America is not as common in many other societies. Some feelings, such as shame, that in Europe are attributed to one's inner state are attributed to external circumstances in other communities.[133] The differences in experiencing and expressing emotions are reflected in the manifestation of common mental disorders, particularly through the different faces of depression and anxiety and their remote masks, somatization and dissociation.

9.1 Depression and Anxiety

Depression has existed in all cultures and ages, and—unlike schizophrenia—since antiquity. Described on ancient papyruses, clay plates, and in the Old Testament, it has been defined with amazing precision (even from the viewpoint of modern classifications) and laconicism by Hippocrates in his 23rd aphorism. The first substantial work on depression, *Tractate on Melancholy*, by Isaac Ibn Omran appeared in the 9th century during the blossoming of Arab medicine under the Abbasid dynasty, while in the 13th century the great Arab physician Maimonides successfully cured the Sultan Saladin's son of his melancholy using psychotherapy—but not herbs or other medicines—because he saw the roots of the illness in the boy's character.[14] Centuries later in Christian Europe, R. Burton's *The Anatomy of Melancholy* in 1621(Fig. 13) not only described the condition in detail,[166] but also left a mark on its further philosophical interpretation in the European intellectual tradition for centuries, endorsing the Eurocentric dichotomy of spirit and body. This dichotomy is one of the main reasons for cultural differences in the physical signs of emotional illness.

Depression and anxiety are presented together because of their obvious overlap and connection. Depression or dysthymia exists in 45.6 % of patients with anxiety disorders in the general practice, and vice versa—51.8 % of patients with depression have an anxiety disorder.[113] Their overlap increases along with their clinical similarity, reaching 67 % between dysthymia and generalized anxiety: both conditions are not intense, but chronic, with common symptoms and underlying neurotic dynamics. Depression and anxiety have biological markers in common, as well as social and comorbidity profiles, and in treatment they respond to the same class of medicines. Such an overlap does not indicate comorbidity, but rather their belonging to a broader spectrum in which the syndromes' key emotions are located on a temporal continuum: current pain (sadness) and future pain (fear).

A certain diagnostic hierarchy exists between them: the lowest level consists of the non-specific *minor* emotional illness[180]—with mild anxiety, depression, and somatization symptoms—numerous in general practice and below diagnostic thresholds, the majority of which are not diseases at all but rather homeostatic responses to environmental stressors, remitting without treatment; above them are the anxiety disorders; and the highest rank within the diagnostic hierarchy of this spectrum is occupied by the full-blown clinical picture of major depression. For this reason, anxiety can be viewed as an underdeveloped form of depression, as its less specific and initial form, or at least as its subvariant.[214] Negative emotionality is shared by both syndromes—combined with the lack of positive

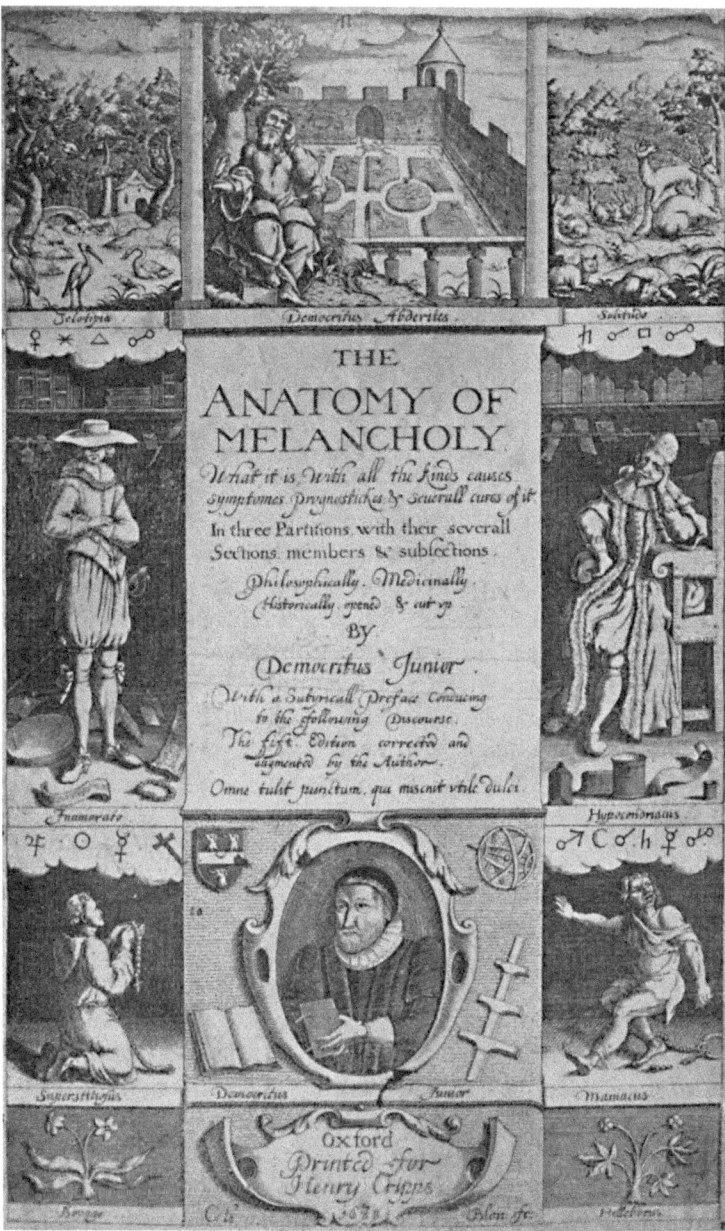

Fig. 13: The Anatomy of Melancholy by R. Burton, 1628 edition (Courtesy to Getty Images)

emotionality in depression and autonomous symptoms in anxiety. The assumption that disguised anxiety plays a role in many of the physical symptoms of depression makes it possible to speak about masked anxiety through an analogy with so-called masked depression.[164]

Unipolar depression is one of the leading causes of years lost to disability (the World Bank indicator of dysfunction due to disease), accounting for 11.9 % of global disabilities.[180] The cost of illness due to all brain diseases in Europe is 798 billion euros, one third of which is attributed to the most common mental disorders: affective disorders—113.4 billion, anxiety disorders—74.4 billion, somatoform disorders—21.2 billion, and headaches—43.5 billion.[152] In these cases, indirect costs make up the majority of the total cost to a higher degree than other diseases when they are compared. The cost of mental illness and the burden of indirect costs outside of wealthier regions of the world is unknown. The scope of the disorders, however, is better understood.

The average values of global prevalence rates disguise, in fact, huge variations in the distribution of common mental disorders in different populations to a much more pronounced extent than schizophrenia. The most comprehensive study by the WHO on the epidemiology of these disorders, with direct interviewing of 85,052 individuals from the general population in 17 countries in Africa, Asia, North and South America, Europe, and the Middle East using the Composite International Diagnostic Interview (CIDI), finds the variation of lifetime prevalence for anxiety disorders to be 4.8–31.0 %, for affective disorders between 3.3 and 21.4 %, and for other common mental disorders from 12.0 to 47.4 %.[113] The predicted lifetime risk is highest in countries with civil unrest, like Israel, Nigeria, and South Africa. A common finding across all cultures is that the onset of anxiety disorders usually occurs quite early, in childhood.

A large meta-analysis of 174 studies in 63 countries,[196] controlling for plenty of variables, shows that 17.6 % of all people have had some common mental disorder in the past year, and that 29.2 % had experienced this at some time in their lives. Women everywhere have higher rates for affective disorders (7. 3 % vs. 4.0 % of men) and anxiety disorders (8.7 % vs. 4.3 % of men). East Asian countries bear significantly lower annual rates and lifetime prevalence, countries in sub-Saharan Africa also have markedly lower annual rates, and these rates are the highest in English-speaking countries worldwide. Against the background of this global picture, the results from some isolated regions like the highest parts of the Andes are surprising. There, an unparalleled frequency of moderate and severe depression of 60 % (28 % moderate and 32 % severe)[224] is found, with the feasible interpretation of non-pathological responses to daily stress through complaining in the "nervios" style which is habitual for the culture (Chapter 11).

Depression is also more common in some closed communities and religious cults, such as the Amish in the USA or Pentecostals, who forbid the expression of aggression and sexual freedom. Suicides are, as a rule, more uncommon in traditional communities, and there are some places where they are virtually unknown. The population specifics of mania are difficult to detect because of its relative rarity and problematic distinction from infectious organic brain syndromes in the Third World.

The dualism between body and spirit in the Western tradition generates difficulties in recognizing and understanding emotional illness in non-Western cultures, where this division does not exist. It is manifest in the diagnostic criteria that go into the formulation of psychological and physical symptoms. The very conceptualization of emotion outside of the physical body is a problem in many traditional cultures where these cohabitate in fusion. The experience of one's identity and the locus of emotions is different in collectivistic communities. The vocabulary is also different. Some languages lack denominations for emotional nuances: words like guilt, shame, or sin have different associations from these in the Judeo-Christian world, while words for anguish or despair (like the Chinese *you-yu*) are associated with different physiological states; in many linguistic families of North America, Africa, and Southeast Asia, there is no word like depression, repression, or depressive as an adjective for mood.[4, 5, 133, 142] Depression (from the Latin, "keep down") in the European view originates from the allegory of a downward direction of one's emotions. The above mentioned linguistic families have an equivalent which means *empty*, i.e., a melancholic person does not suffer from depressed emotions, but is devoid of them.

The expression of emotions is subject to folk customs and rules in both sickness and health. In some communities, like those of New Guinea and among the Yanomami people of Brazil, dramatic outbursts of anger are frequently demonstrated, while others, such as Inuit communities and in Tahiti, very rarely show anger; the expression of sadness is encouraged by some (e.g., Iranians) and banned by others (e.g., Navajo Indians).[173, 181] Similar distinctions also exist among different social layers and subcultures, for instance among educated, wealthy citizens and those who inhabit the ghettos of the same cities. The narrative of complaining is multifaceted. What people choose to share depends on their view about what is socially and situationally acceptable. In many cultures, people describe heat, a lump, stone, or ball, scrawling, twisting, burning, pinching, itching, pulling, throbbing, ringing, or exploding, instead of emotions. Their complaints are usually consonant with beliefs about their causes. In general, somatization masks and metaphors are more common in traditional cultures, especially in Africa, Latin America, the Middle East, and Southeast

Asia, as well as among immigrants from these places, and in some places even include a tendency to cluster organs and systems such as guts (Japan), muscles, skin, etc. Certain cultural differences also concern the key symptom of depression, anhedonia, despite its usual association with biological markers such as hyperactivity in the left ventro-median prefrontal cortex.

Clinical case. A 48-year-old male *pomak* (a Muslim of Balkan origin, or *ahryanin*), married with three children, a cattle breeder, had for months been restless, gloomy, incessantly sighing noisily and complaining of an unbearable heat in his chest, comparing it to live coals; he was constantly underdressed and sweating, even in cold weather, losing weight and unable to sleep unless he drank some *rakiya* (a traditional Bulgarian spirit). He continued to adequately care for his cattle and experience pleasure, particularly upon seeing his youngest grandson, and denied feeling sadness, despair, or any other kind of depressive affect. Twenty-five years earlier, he had suffered from abundant sweating for about a year without any other complaints, feeling ashamed of the odor of his sweat, especially in front of women, and for this reason secluding himself. During the new crisis, he was treated with high doses of antidepressants from different classes without effect, but with even greater agitation and the emergence of suicidal plans. Ten procedures of electro-convulsive therapy (ECT) brought about no result. Improvement did occur after the application of maximal doses of maprotiline, which he continued to take for 15 years afterwards, though in lower doses and combined with lithium, without relapse. The patient has refused to reduce his dosage or stop taking the medicine.

This case displays rather typical behavior for emotional illnesses in this closed minority subculture. When admitted in the clinic, a half-ironic diagnostic exercise was conducted by post-graduate trainees with instructions to literally apply the diagnostic criteria. The patient was assessed according to the ICD-10 and the DSM-IV as formally meeting criteria for generalized anxiety disorder and somatization disorder, however, without entirely fulfilling the criteria for major depression. Nevertheless, the trainees were certain that the patient should be treated for major depression. His severe agitation, serious risk of suicide, and treatment responses were not only evidence for the depressive nature of the episode, but also left no doubt about its severity and treatment resistance, including the unusual ECT resistance. The absence of anhedonia and distinct depressive affect, as well as undisturbed daily functioning, contrasted the syndrome's severity and introduced an atypicality that may suggest analogy with a mixed state in the course, although the patient had never experienced mania or hypomania and his personality profile was clearly introverted. Sweating is a peculiar but common ethno-physiological characteristic of discomfort, and its perception and interpretation had also been inserted into the patient's morbid view of the world: e.g., being caused by "live coals", the odor of the sweat causing shame in the past. The idea of emitting unpleasant odor may reach a more delusional conviction and serve as a motive for suicide, while shame—not guilt—is the key emotion of depression in this traditional community. The patient's behavior during follow-up treatment was also characteristic: a preoccupation with protection against relapse, over-compliance, especially with biological treatment, and over-treatment.

As compared to the relatively stable factor structure of schizophrenia in different cultures (Chapter 8), factor analyses of depression and anxiety in different populations have produced extremely multifaceted and unstable factors which tautologically reproduce the style of illness behavior and complaints by statistical clustering. A constant finding is the representation of physical and psychological symptoms on separate factors in developed countries, and their merging into a common factor in the developing world.[142] This is more in unison with a more holistic view about the body and the mental world in health and illness found in traditional cultures than with the Eurocentric dualistic mentality.

The search for the syndrome structure of depression via factor analysis and its connection with culture is often based on a simple view of the syndrome as being homogenous, and having a horizontal disposition of symptoms: x available from y of the checklist. The fact that 14 factors, without links between them, have been isolated shows the many-sided nature of depression. It appears in different conditions, just like inflammation syndrome in general medicine. As with inflammation, depression too may have different causes and play different roles in pathological reactions and processes. For this reason, it is much more appropriate to speak about depressions rather than depression. The clinical diversity is so large that it is possible for two patients with depression to have not even one symptom in common, despite sharing a common diagnosis: e.g., low mood, motor retardation, feelings of guilt, weight loss, and early awakening in one of them, with irritability, agitation, poor concentration, and difficulty falling asleep in the other. Hereditary factors are very heterogeneous, significant life events and personality pathologies are rules rather than exceptions, and treatment responses are so incredibly diverse, especially in moderate and mild depressions, that general guidelines must be ignored at the expense of developing target treatments for the subtypes according to individual profiles. Deconstructing the syndrome shows its inner structure, not along a horizontal axis, but in a hierarchical and in-depth way.

Deficits in drives, such as low energy and libido, and changes in sleep, appetite, and weight encompass the deepest level of impairment; they are also

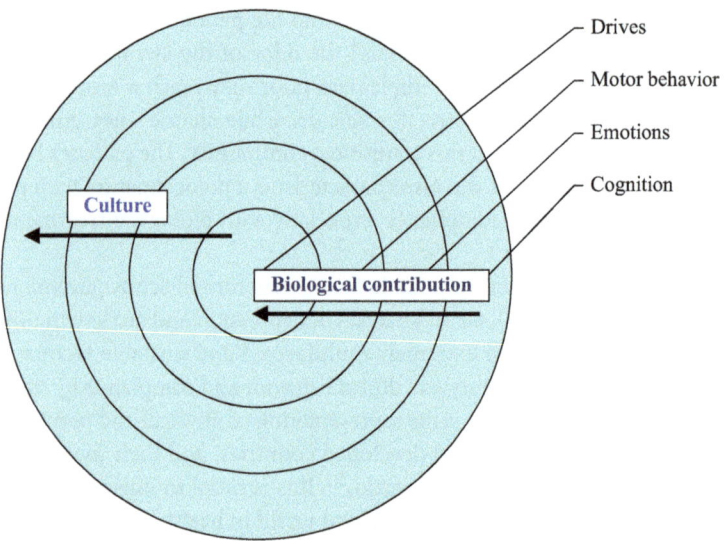

Fig. 14: Deconstruction of the depressive syndrome

probably influenced by a circadian dysregulation, leading to large geographical differences in these manifestations according to annual hours of sunlight. Above them are changes in motor behavior: retardation, uneasiness, and agitation. Mood changes follow next: gloominess, anhedonia, suicidality, and anxiety; and are supervened by an outer layer of cognitive disturbance: poor concentration, retarded tempo, low motivation, memory deficit, apathia, executive dysfunction, ruminations, and guilt. This model allows for the distinction to be made between cultural and biological contributions to the syndrome. The influence of culture increases from the core to the periphery (despite cultural differences within the core due to geographical differences). On the contrary, biological contributions increase from the periphery to the core (Fig. 14). The probability of success for biological treatments also increases in this direction (with ECT being the most effective in deep impairment), which explains their lack of effectiveness in mild syndromes with only emotional and cognitive manifestations.

Depressiveness in Mexicans and Iranians is frequently displayed through hostility toward other family members.[181] And yet anxiety in Latin America usually manifests with the pattern of *susto* and *ataque de nervios*, which are considered to be culture specific syndromes (Chapter 11) but in fact constitute culturally accepted illness models of common mental disorders. The recognition of clinically expressed depression among Hopi Indians and Puerto Ricans, two populations where average general depressiveness is salient,[145] requires the diagnostic threshold for depression to shift according to the population norm—an example of the necessity to "calibrate" clinical units of measurement against the context. The upheld (from the ICD-9) category of neurasthenia in China unites the common combination of anxious, depressive, and somatoform symptoms in a professionally and culturally acceptable way, thus excluding irrelevant comorbidity and interpretations of different models of illness behavior.

Minor emotional illnesses can be trivialized down to commonly accepted styles of expression in societies with high levels of uncertainty avoidance and greater power distance, where the fatalistic view that personal fortune does not depend on personal efforts is popular and behaviors such as not assuming personal responsibility, complaining, and self-pity are encouraged. Verbalization and the topic of complaints are less informative than are emotional expressiveness and its context. In the words of Nietzsche, "thoughts are the shadows of our feelings—always darker, emptier and simpler". A culturally competent clinical assessment of common mental disorders should account for the means of perceiving distress and problems in patients' subcultures, explanatory models of illness (such as bewitchment or physiological dysfunction), prevailing idioms of behavioral illness (such as falling down, obsessive doubts, or punishing oneself for not using licensed programs by breaking a computer), the roles these idioms play out in the community (such as indicating sickness or being cursed), relevant diagnostic categories, and the degree of deterioration of functioning.

9.2 Somatization and Dissociation

The conceptualization of somatization as the presence of physical symptoms without physical disease is problematic for many reasons, one of which is uncertainty regarding the absence of somatic disease. There are many functional somatic disturbances without any overt pathologies or certain psychological involvement. The idea of somatization as a way to express distress or internal conflict is culture specific in itself, belonging to patterns of Western thinking about neurotic symptom formation which began in the 19th century. Somatization has kaleidoscopic manifestations in depressive and anxiety disorders, but it is also found in other diseases, e.g., in the prodromes of schizophrenia, and forms a separate diagnostic category only when it is not due to another pathology. In the DSM-5,[6] this category has already been changed to *somatic symptom* disorder, a name that emphasizes its phenomenology without making any guesses about its underlying mechanism, as implied by denominations like somatization and somatoform.

This is a heterogeneous group overlapping with the depression-anxiety spectrum, as well as with culturally normative behaviors. Somatization manifestations may not be signs of illness at all. There is cultural variety even in the physical symptoms, such as complaints common in Southeast Asia that sperm is present in the urine, or burning and itching of the head in Africa.[145, 208] In societies with strong traditional beliefs and a strict social order and norms, some ideas might be so rigidly held that they hamper distinctions from being made between an anxious preoccupation with physical symptoms and hypochondriac delusion, resulting in the attribution of delusional characteristics to nonpsychotic hypochondriasis from different cultures.

Idiosyncratic manifestations of somatization are usually described as culture specific syndromes (Chapter 11), although their designation as pure somatization is problematic. Koro syndrome, for instance, combines anxiety, hypochondriasis, and dysmorphophobia, but may be psychotic too. Similarly, sensations of malaise in the head in Nigeria and *shinkeishitsu* in Japan are more closely related to Chinese neurasthenia than to somatization disorder because they are both mixed anxiety-depressive states with somatic signs.

Dissociation is an archaic and universal manifestation, although its presumed mechanism—the *dissociation* of the idea–emotion complex along with removing unacceptable impulses, thoughts, or feelings from the consciousness—is also a culturally specific product of Western thinking. In traditional communities where the requirement for individual self-control and self-observation is weak (as compared to collective control and observation), a change in consciousness with blanks in personal experience and memories can be achieved more easily. When it is part of normative rituality, the change occurs spontaneously with either absent or minimal psychopathology, or through a conscious search with the aid of self-absorption or psychoactive drugs.

Both dissociation and somatization need some suggestibility and inclination toward a narrowed consciousness which causes one to either focus on a sensation (somatization) or detach from some aspects of reality or the self (dissociation). The most common model of dissociation in the Third World is possession by spirits or other supernatural forces (Chapter 7). Trance possession states, from a cultural point of view, are universal rather than specific: they have been part of diverse cult practices for millennia, though they differ in the specific details of the subject matter and in folkloric heritage. The basic experience of being possessed by external forces, however, is common and—in its essence—is dissociative. That is why their assignment to culture specific syndromes is misleading.

Possession, as was already described in Chapter 7, can be a normative belief, a dissociative experience, or the content of a symptom in heterogeneous clinical states. The normal or pathological status of possession, and its nosological affiliation when pathological, is subject to case-by-case judgment according to the deterioration of functioning, not by cultural stereotypes.

If dissociation is a response to traumatic experience, then it is obviously subject to strong cultural influences because the symptoms' content reflects various traumatic experiences, albeit through a universal mechanism. The specific dissociative manifestations include aimless running, as in the already non-existent *pibloktoq* among Eskimos or *chakore* in Panama, which is related to a psychogenic fugue state.[145] Amok, also uncommon today, is sometimes included here, however it is more frequent in men, unlike most of the dissociative syndromes (more common in women), and is related to severe homicidal aggression—convincing case descriptions bring it closer to a state of acute psychosis (Chapter 11). Similar, too, are trance-like depersonalizations, a sudden collapse with the loss of sensation and memory in Haitians, and frequent conversion seizures in Indians.[142] Transitional displays of *latah* in South East Asia (Chapter 11), e.g., during funerals, conflicts with mothers-in-law, protests, or other ceremonies, might not be pathological at all. When these displays get out of control and step outside of these circumstances, though, *latah* transforms into pathology, sometimes with the pattern of hyper-acute reactive psychosis. In this case, as in possession, its manifestations lie along a continuum of culturally acceptable behaviors, moving from mild to severe psychopathology. In general, somatization and dissociation are continuums of experiences modeled by culture which can be either normal or pathological. When pathological, the entire account of the overall clinical picture offers reasoning in search of analogies with known categories, in contrast with ascribing them to museum-status "exoticism" as syndromes with special denominations, thus feeding nosologomania and Orwellian *Newspeak* in psychiatry.

10 Abnormal Behaviors and Culture

> There is no dark side of the moon, really.
> Matter of fact, it's all dark.
>
> *Pink Floyd*

The etiology of most abnormal behaviors is unknown, however, the modeling effect of cultural views on abnormality and its culturally-sanctioned manifestation or transformation is obvious. The same pathology may display behavioral alternatives, depending on its interaction with the environment. The prevalence of impulse control disorders varies, for instance, between 0.3 and 25 % of the global population.[113] With clear evidence of a neurobiological substrate of impulse control, such a huge variation—from being extremely rare to affecting one quarter of the general population—is a sign of the different faces of pathology. In cultures that are permissive towards alcohol and drug use, impaired impulse control can manifest itself through abuse and addiction; while in cultures that are restrictive towards drinking and addictive substances, it may acquire the form of angry outbursts or either personality or affective pathologies. We found in a Bulgarian sample that alcohol abuse could be an alternative to borderline personality disorder in a cultural context that is stricter with regard to challenging behaviors than it is to drinking.[155] The peculiar *cultural equivalents* of common underlying pathologies are intrinsic to abnormal behaviors and applicable to anorexia, paraphilias, severe adaptation reactions, and other illness metamorphoses.

10.1 Alcohol and Drugs

The need for intoxication of any kind (euphorization, sedation, or altered consciousness) is timeless and universal. There has never been a pre-historical or developed society where this need was not satisfied with whatever means available. Fermentation was known even to primordial people, but only started to be consciously developed and used after the transition from hunting and gathering to settlement and agriculture some 11,000 years ago in Mesopotamia and the Nile River Valley, where the most ancient of artefacts and written records contain information about the consumption of wine and beer.[50, 211] Distillation and its product, spirits, was an achievement made approximately 10,000 later. In antiquity, in an environment raging with infectious diseases and a shortage of safe drinking water, the favorable effect of alcohol in moderate doses on health was well known. Pliny the Elder recommends moderate use and avoiding any extremes, including total abstention.[131] Avicenna, himself a wine connoisseur, refers to it as "an enemy of drunkards and a friend of wise men".[14]

Alcohol has been intimately woven into daily life, eating, ritual, creativity, sexual behavior, and societal organization in Mediterranean and European civilizations. The perfection of winemaking in the Middle Ages was achieved chiefly by monks in the monastery vineyards and cellars, thus endorsing the link between Christian culture and alcohol—symbolized in the act of the Sacrament. Aphorisms like Faulkner's "Civilization begins with distillation" are excerpts from an age-old series of famous sayings, verses, and fiction which both glorify and ridicule drinking and its consequences found in the Old Testament as well as the works of Homer, Omar Khayyam, Shakespeare, Rabelais, Pushkin, Hasek, Churchill, Steinbeck, Bukowski, and Yerofeyev, among others. One of many possible criteria for classifying cultures is their tolerance to alcohol, i.e., restrictive, ambivalent, or permissive. Although this may appear to be a simplified ascertainment, historically it seems obvious that human progress has prospered in permissive *alcohol* cultures. And this is not a Christian or Eurocentric perspective: the flourishing of the Arab world under the caliphate from the 9th to 12th centuries, for instance, was accompanied by a tolerant attitude towards moderate drinking despite its being banned by the Quran, while the caliphate's subsequent decline bore witness to a more dogmatic obedience to this restriction.

The oldest known psychoactive drug is the poppy seed. Prepared as tea, juice, or in combination with milk or food, it has been used for almost 7,000 years in Sumer, Crete, and Egypt for pain relief, to induce sleep, and for recreational purposes. Hippocrates recommended the practice, and, in some places, the juice was even used to soothe crying babies.[194] The birthplace of the coca plant, as well as peyote (containing raw mescaline), ololiuqui, and different hallucinogenic mushrooms, is Latin America; cannabis and betel originated in Southeast Asia; and khat—in Ethiopia and Yemen. These are the places where *drug trafficking* began. From the Middle East, poppy products spread to Greece, Egypt, China, and India. Smoking opium became especially popular in the Far East. From Southeast Asia, cannabis products known as marijuana, hashish, ganja, bhang, dagga, and other names were transferred to the Middle East and Europe, where they replaced opium. Marijuana and hashish have been used to combat depression and malaria, and as painkillers.[47, 133, 148, 194] Both gained popularity among Arabs[4, 151] and subsequently all Muslims as an alternative to alcohol, banned by

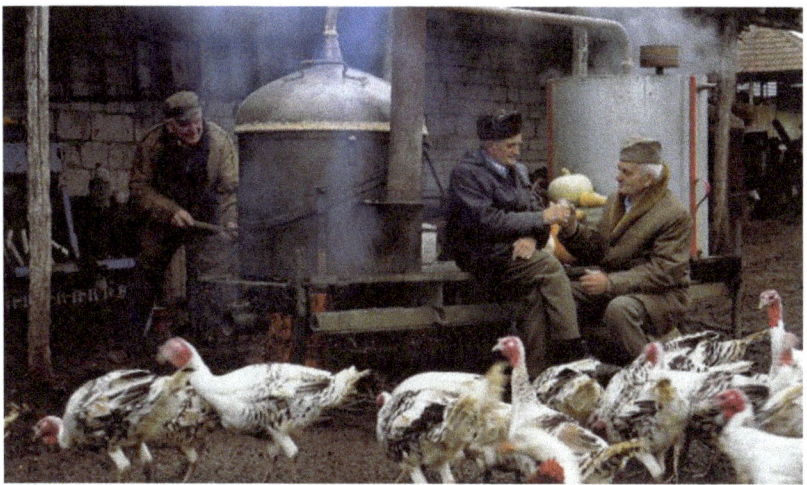

Fig. 15: A rakiya still, the Bulgarian forum

the Quran, accompanied by the argument that, unlike wine, they do not blur the consciousness but move it closer to God.[14, 194]

During the Middle Ages, hashish also became very popular in Europe, and in the post-Columbian era tobacco and coca were brought to the Old World too. In Bulgaria, especially in the northwest, the cultivation of hemp (*grasti*) for knitting ropes and sacks, but also for popularized chewing and smoking, was carried out on a mass scale under Ottoman rule. In the global migration of drugs, examples such as khat and betel have only appeared locally. After being synthesized at the turn of the 20th century for medical purposes, cocaine has been used on an increasingly large scale, while barbiturate addiction, a major health and social problem in Europe and America throughout the 20th century, appears to have been a transitory epidemic and has practically disappeared. LSD's popularity rose in the 1960s, decreasing in the following decades in favor of the growing prevalence of amphetamines, phencyclidine, and designer drugs.

The frequency of alcohol's pathologic use is not precisely known, and it has natural distinctions between cultures. In Europe, the cradle of the civilization breastfed by alcohol (Fig. 15), 55 million persons today exhibit "alcohol irresponsible behavior", according to the WHO's reserved expression, and some 23 million are estimated to be alcohol dependent.[131] Regardless of the increase in total alcohol use, the portion of spirits consumed in Europe after World War II decreased while the consumption of beverages with a lower percentage of alcohol, mainly beer and wine, were on the rise. The annual cost of illnesses due to addictions in Europe is 65.7 billion euros,[152] with a high portion accounting for indirect costs. The prevalence of all drug addictions (a preferred term, as not all substances have strictly psychoactive effects) in different regions of the world is between 1.3 and 15 %.[113] The current prevalence in different cultures may vary from zero to first or second place among all mental disorders. It is higher in men (on average, 7.5 % vs. 2 % in women)[113] everywhere, but the disparity in this ratio is greater in many societies—anywhere from 2:1 to 40:1—for one and the same drug. Some regions of Southeast Asia where betel chewing is more common among women are the exception to this rule.

A study involving 43,092 individuals in the USA found a 17.8 % lifetime and 4.7 % 12-month prevalence rate of alcohol abuse; those rates were 12.5 % and 3.8 %, respectively, for alcohol dependence;[81] and both abuse and dependence were higher in five groups: men, whites, Native Americans, and unmarried and low-income individuals. Only 24.1 % of alcohol-dependent participants in this study had ever been treated, and when controlled for other variables, any link with the abuse of other drugs, affective and anxiety disorders, and personality pathology was weak. This important finding shows that comorbidity, which accounts for the mechanical and horizontal coexistence of different syndromes, is overestimated. In fact, the finding reflects the affective and anxiety manifestations of alcohol's multifaceted pathology, not comorbidity.

The pathological use of alcohol and drugs is, to some extent, proportional to their per capita consumption; the link, however, is not at all a linear one. In permissive alcohol cultures, like those of the Mediterranean, moderate drinking is very common, yet pathological use makes up a relatively low share of general consumption. In ambivalent cultures, like Scandinavia and Ireland, though drinking is not as common, pathological use and its complications are disproportionally high as compared to general consumption. Globally, alcohol use is highest in Europe, while problems related to alcohol use are most frequent in Eastern Europe and Russia and are least common in Africa. Alcohol consumption is higher among Orthodox Christians, Catholics, and Liberal Protestants; it is lower in Conservative Protestants (such as Evangelists and Adventists), Muslims, and Buddhists. The ratio between alcohol dependent persons who are known to health care services and the entire population of alcohol dependent persons is estimated at approximately 1:10—for drug addiction, this ratio is approximately 1:3,[194]—with vast differences according to the social environment and the availability of addiction treatment services.

The diagnoses of abuse and dependence have high reliability and validity, despite problems related to the identification, restriction and encouragement of use by ethnic or subcultural environments. Pathological use may not seem pathological if the environment supports it, e.g., in "bottle gangs", particularly in Native Americans.[145] Vice versa, even minor consumption of alcohol or coffee may be perceived as pathological by others, e.g., Mormons. Conforming entirely to the attitudes of the subculture is misleading and results in relativism towards diagnostic rules. Every type of use is risky or pathological if it is associated with increased tolerance (e.g., drinking more than 10 drinks daily without signs of heavy intoxication), or considerable risk (e.g., using marijuana when piloting an aircraft), even if supported by the individual's subculture. Ethnic or cultural norms of use are not themselves part of the criteria for pathological use. The scope and the style of drinking or drug use are undoubtedly related to the environment, however, the pathology itself is far more universal. Unlike other mental disorders, abuse and dependence syndromes have biological markers: symptoms of intoxication and withdrawal, organic states (like dementia), evidence of use (e.g., urinalysis for cannabis or a blood alcohol test), and evidence of physical harm (e.g., heightened liver enzymes or increased volume of corpuscular erythrocytes). The typology of alcoholism by Lesch, combining biological, intrapsychic, and environmental criteria, is an empirical one which has been reproduced so far in every population where it has been tested.[131]

Pathophysiological changes are common across cultures, albeit with qualitative distinctions according to the style of usage. In ambivalent cultures, such as Ireland, drinking is rarer, limited predominantly to weekends, and associated mainly with consuming spirits, leading to severe intoxications with frequent injuries, violence, confrontations with law enforcement, and a high risk for cardio-vascular diseases. Drinking in tolerant cultures like France is continuous, but more controlled, and mainly consists of wine, not leading to severe intoxications (nor to full sobriety), social problems, or injuries; still, it does cause more frequent gastro-intestinal problems and liver damage. Other common and sustainable features are early onset in all cultures, usually in adolescence and early adulthood, and the average term from the onset of dependence to the first contact for treatment is 10 years for alcohol, 3 for heroin, and 1 for cocaine.[142]

The more restrictive a culture is towards alcohol and drug use, the more conspicuous is the role of personality pathology, heredity, and family use in its rise. Some demographic groups, such as children and teens growing up in ghettos, and clinical ones, like people in organic states who cannot tolerate the effects of even minor doses, are especially vulnerable to pathological use. The qualitative WHO limits for safe drinking should indeed be considered as relative due to huge differences in alcohol tolerance on an individual level and across populations. The Caucasian race has the highest tolerance, probably due to the natural selection of liver enzymes in the millennia-long history of drinking. Personal measure also plays an important role in the assessing quantities. A clinician who is a heavy drinker may ignore any levels below their own (this is the basis for the anecdotal saying that an alcoholic is someone who drinks more than his or her doctor). And, vice versa, a physician who is a teetotaler, or drinks very rarely, may identify risky or pathological drinking in anyone who exceeds their personal limits. These subjective norms operate, just like every cultural sanction, unconsciously and relatively independently of the physician's cognitive competence concerning addiction.

Familial and social problems associated with pathological use also vary according to cultural affiliation. Secretive drinking, stocking up on alcohol, and drinking alone, for instance, are all much more common among white members of the middle class than in minority groups. The use of even very low doses of alcohol or other substances, while totally acceptable in other cultural contexts, may result in community detachment and even rejection in restrictive communities such as Adventists, the Amish, Quakers, or other conservative denominations. Treatment approaches also differ according to the context, especially according to one's physical health and access to a supportive social network, family, home, or job, and require separate algorithms depending on the lines of distinction based on these characteristics.

10.2 Personality and Behavioral Pathologies

The pathology of personality is an extension of the diversity of personalities. Generally, it is more prevalent in individualistic cultures which prioritize autonomy and individual norms than it is in traditional communities. The prevalence of personality disorders in the general population is between 1 and 3 % for each of them, and between 10 and 13 % for all of them in total, but in many regions, especially rural ones in the Third World, it is unknown.[5] Out of all mental disorders, the portion of indirect costs of illness is the highest in personality pathologies.[152] The theoretical prediction of the probability of combining extremities on Cloninger's temperamental dimensions[40]—novelty seeking, reward dependence, harm avoidance, and persistence—produces an average result of 2 % for each combination of abnormal traits. The coincidence of this result with empirically derived rates, as well as the hypothesis that these behaviors are mediated in each dimension by a specific neurotransmitter, are arguments for a biological contribution to personality pathologies, or at least to their temperamental component.

This contribution is also supported by the links between some personality disorders and diseases such as schizotypal-schizophrenia, paranoid-paranoid psychosis, borderline-bipolar disorder and drug abuse, and avoidant-depression and anxiety disorders. Personality disorders share common neurophysiological mechanisms and psychological defenses both with their healthy prototypes and illness analogues; for this reason, they may be viewed as a transition between the norm and pathology, a *forme fruste* of the mental illness which escalates these common mechanisms and defenses from health to pathology. On a conditional axis between biological and socio-cultural poles, the personality disorder types can be arranged in the following order: schizotypal, antisocial, schizoid, borderline, paranoid, histrionic, avoidant, anankastic, and dependent.

The manifestation of some personality traits at the expense of others is encouraged by cultural contexts[37, 38] and child-rearing practices. Traits like assertiveness, boldness, and independence are desired in many societies when forming boys' characters, but are considered shortcomings by some Native Americans, who rather stimulate traits like submissiveness and passivity—resembling the prototype of a dependent personality.[102] In smaller communities with more traditional values, general norms are well integrated on a personal level and abnormalities of personality are not dramatically conspicuous, while in larger communities with a diversity of values that frequently compete with one another, norms are not rigid and may not be very well integrated individually—additionally, abnormal behaviors may be more conspicuous. The main types of personality pathologies are indeed probably universal for most societies (excepting rural regions) but the norm against which they deviate is different. Anthropological investigations of a conditionally typical personality for different communities[102, 181] demonstrate the cultural relativity of prevailing personality profiles and constructed community norms. The impairment of functioning in different spheres is a mandatory diagnostic criterion for personality disorder, while the norms of functioning and deviation in the same spheres are cultural.

Examples of traits which are phenomenologically part of the pathology of personality, but may or may not be dysfunctional, depending on the environment, are present in all personality disorders. Mistrustfulness, uncovering threats, and believing in evil eyes and curses are common in some Mediterranean communities, and at the same time are paranoid personality disorder traits. The schizoid characteristics of extreme reticence, refusal of pleasure and indifference to the external world are actually fundamental tenets of some Buddhist monks and ascetics from other religious denominations and cults, while the schizotypal conceptions of magic and odd perceptions, appearance, and beliefs can be attributed to shamans and mystical leaders of closed communities. Antisocial traits are more common in the ghettos of large metropoles; histrionic ones—among actors, models, and members of show business; narcissistic traits—among successful businesspeople and political leaders; anxious or dependent personalities are more frequently encountered in underprivileged and poor communities; and anankastic ones—among priests, scientists, and craftspeople such as jewelers or watchmakers. In the same way that an individual with a personality disorder is a caricature of otherwise normal, but extreme, human characteristics, so too this person, like a caricature, reflect the subculture of his or her origin.

Eating disorders are directly related to cultural norms regarding a slender figure and attitudes towards eating. Anorexia is frequently given as an example that is culturally specific to Western societies—where being thin is perceived as possessing beauty, sex appeal, and success. Genuine anorexia nervosa is, in fact, rare even in developed countries, with an approximate prevalence of just 1 in 1000,[142] and this is why many epidemiological surveys do not include it in their analyses.[113] New research shows that the disorder is probably unrecognized and underestimated in different minorities. In the USA, where it is estimated to have the highest prevalence, anorexia and bulimia among white college students affect 4 % of men and 13 % of women, while among black students they affect 2 % of men and 3 % of women.[142] The fear of gaining weight may be absent or unpronounced in minorities, despite the other criteria for anorexia being met. As with white patients, minorities with anorexia and bulimia come from elevated social classes. In Asia, eating disorders are found only in large cities and in families from higher social circles.[119] Surveys that identify eating disorders in minority communities and immigrants from traditional cultures in developed countries,[142] in fact, reflect an overall submission to pressure for acculturation rather than the authentic cultures of their origin. In my own practice in a very traditional culture in Africa, I never never encountered a local case of anorexia nervosa (nor obsessive-compulsive disorder or suicide attempts). Self-imposed starvation for the sake of appearances is totally incomprehensible in areas with a shortage of food.

The fear of gaining weight, or its absence, is frequently explained by cultural specificity (this fear is also characteristic to women without anorexia in the Western world), and by cultural comparisons (black women, at least in the United States, are more overweight than white women), thus even going so far as to suggest that the fear diagnostic criterion for anorexia should be dropped for minorities. This criterion, however, is connected with the eating disorder's core disturbance—a disturbed self-perception of body image—and its exclusion brings into question whether genuine anorexia can be diagnosed, or if the patient's loss of weight could be due to other causes, e.g., depression. Eastern cultures have strict, ancient traditions of control over food, eating, and their importance to one's appearance and health.[133, 138] In China, where the notion of beauty is focused mainly on the face and not the body, anorexia is frequently precipitated by the appearance of acne. At the same time, anorexia is universally less frequent in men, yet has a poorer course, particularly if it is the prodrome of another mental disorder (as with the clinical case in Chapter 6).

The description and interpretation of sexual behavior disorders should also take into account the sexual practices which are tolerated by cultures. Moralistic dogmas, particularly of the major religions, limit sexual activity to its reproductive function, condemning virtually all other forms and manifestations. In a moralistic hierarchy, sex is a destructive force that has to be controlled not only by personal responsibility, but also in a punitive social framework. For this reason, religious orthodoxy is at the core of most sexual dysfunctions in men. Sexual dysfunctions in behavior are present in different cultures, however, they do not everywhere meet the criteria for pathologies due to the diagnostic requirement that such behavior causes distress, which is not always the case. The experience of distress in developed societies is frequently associated with high performance expectations and with the notion of an orgasm being a mandatory part of the act. In some cultures, premature ejaculation is not perceived to be problem,[208] and in others the focus on genital sex and the role of the male erection is absent. Social distinctions, like women from lower social classes experiencing orgasms less frequently than those from the upper class, are also found.

Cultural stereotypes impose standards for attractiveness and sexual performance that may be experienced as traumatic by individuals for whom they are unrealistic. Stereotypes about the machismo of Latin Americans, with the saint-whore antinomy in their attitudes towards women and the ritual eroticizing of some behaviors, as well as other stereotypes about the hyper sexuality of people from African descent, may cause real sexual dysfunctions because of the anxiety caused by being unable to live up to these notions, internalized as they might be.

According to some anthropologists, paraphilia emerges as a substitutive practice in societies where easy access to a partner is lacking, and the only way to discharge sexual energy is masturbation.[142] These practices are not regarded as pathological everywhere; in some communities, for instance, pedophilia is still assumed to be natural and acceptable behavior. According to the Sunni hadiths, Aisha, the last wife of the Prophet Muhammad, married him when she was 7 years old, although the marriage was allegedly not consummated until she reached the age of 9,[114] and at 18 she was already a widow. Some Buddhist monks develop formicophilia—the pleasure experienced from crawling insects or nails being placed over the genitalia. The ancient Daoist belief that the retention of sperm is healthy does not correlate the male orgasm with ejaculation, and lies at the core of different behaviors which control sex by postponing climax to the greatest extent possible. Despite the presence of a sexual connotation, koro and dhat are not sexual dysfunctions but are, rather, culture specific syndromes with anxious, depressive, and dysmorphophobic characteristics (Chapter 11)—nonetheless, they are usually accompanied by impotence or premature ejaculation.

Different gender identities have been described in different cultures prior to the contemporary proliferation of these identities corresponding to the two main biological sexes. The polymorphic cultures of Polynesia have more fluid identities,[47] not strictly male or female but with traits from both of them, however fluctuating towards one or the other according to life stage and social status. Several genders are also recognized among some tribes of North America and the Chukchi of Siberia.

Cultural differences in stress and adaptation reactions are expressed through a spectrum of non-specific somatization and anxiety manifestations (Chapter 9), with "loss of face", shame, and depressiveness. It is assumed that the high prevalence of unipolar depression is due to adaptation disturbances.[142] They are defined by the exclusion of other mental disorders, which in turn categorizes them hierarchically at the lowest rank. Despite this, the role of these categories will increase alongside the cultural transposition of large masses of people, which includes increasing numbers of immigrants and refugees. Although stressors and their perception are modeled by cultural experience and attitudes, some of the most severe stressors—like murder and torture—are universal, and come with universally severe reactions.

11 Culture Specific Syndromes

> Nothing in Zanzibar is as it seems.
>
> Dr. D. Livingstone

The designation "culture specific" is imprecise, because all psychiatric syndromes, even the organic ones, have their cultural specifics. In this provisional entity, transcultural psychiatry traditionally includes syndromes united only by the uncertain presumption that they are present in one culture, while uncommon in others. It is debatable which syndromes should be included here because there are innumerable nuances and variations. These states are exotic, ethnographic local behavioral idioms that reconstruct their meaning, which may seem obscure to the external observer, from the local cosmogony. They are also called psychogenic, hysterical, ethnic, or exotic psychoses, or culture bound, or culture reactive, syndromes.[142, 145, 158] Schizophrenia and affective disorders, despite their marked cultural differences (sometimes to the extent of unrecognizability and diagnostic confusion), are universally known and accessible for examination with the so-called *etic* approach. Unlike them, and in favor of relativism, culture specific syndromes are evidence of cultural uniqueness and can be understood through the so-called *emic* approach (Chapter 5).

Whether these are indeed unique syndromes, formed by specific combinations of cultural heredity and peculiarities of biological isolates and climate, or variants of common syndromes, though significantly transformed by the abovementioned factors, is unknown. The combination between culture, biology, and geographical specifics in each of them is different, with each of these factors bearing a different relative weight. For this reason, their assignment to common categories or larger entities, such as psychogenic and organic, is more acceptable for some syndromes but is simultaneously irrelevant for others.

Their incomprehensibility to the external observer makes any attempts at interpretation, which do not take into account the ethnographic and qualitative research immersion in the local cultural context inappropriate. A more adequate metaphor to use here would be understanding culture as the perception of taste, e.g., tasting wine, as opposed to the rational research approach. An experienced sommelier can describe wine with different qualities (strength, color, substance, ripeness, aroma, ratio between fruit and oak, acidity, tannins), but the bouquet of senses is richer than verbal expression. It is only possible to probe deeply into the specific aspects of some cultures, and as external observation might not catch some essential yet particularly indescribable traits, it is often misleading. Due to this, the great explorer of Africa Dr. Livingstone, mesmerized by the magical charm of Zanzibar and its aura of indolence and unreality, wrote that "nothing is as it seems" there. In its colonial context, this expression is frequently referred to as much less allegorical than it seems—especially in combination with large quantities of gin, heat and malaria. Culture specific syndromes are mostly said to be found in cultures where taboos play a role in concealing much from the outside observer.

The ontological status of these syndromes is problematic. Primarily, it is not clear how they are distinguishable from other psychiatric syndromes which have been described and established in the discipline according to European and American traditions—making them *culturally specific* in the eyes of the rest of the world. This Eurocentric approach refers to "exotic" syndromes from the Third World, those that are not known in developed countries, as culture specific. From the viewpoint of developing nations, however, many common pathologies in Europe and North America are themselves culture specific because they do not exist in the Third World. Anorexia, bulimia, and obsessive-compulsive disorder are totally unknown in traditional communities where food, staring at the female figure (if it is not entirely covered),[5] or folk prototypes of obsessions are either rare or absent. At the same time, these have already become noticeable in some communities and metropoles of the Third World that are subject to accelerated secular transitions and cultural change. Alcoholism is a peculiar culture specific syndrome, deeply rooted in the Judeo-Christian tradition, while in the rest of the world alcohol is either unknown or banned in public spaces. The same also applies to gambling and so-called type A behavior patterns, characterized by ambitiousness, heart disease, a constant shortage of time, workaholism, competitiveness, and aggressiveness.

Hwa-byung. This has been identified in Korea, and among Korean immigrants, mostly in the USA. The main symptoms are stomach pain, burning sensations, and a resultant fear of death; these are frequently accompanied by tiredness, accelerated breathing, insomnia, lack of appetite, muscle pain, and other discomfort. *Byung* means illness in Korean, while *hwa* translates to anger or fire. In traditional Asian beliefs, fire is one of the basic elements of the culturally structured reality. Illness occurs when there are imbalances or inharmonious relations between these elements, in this case an excess of fire. Excessive anger, according to Korean folk healers, can precipitate many diseases. Descriptions of specific cases of this syndrome commonly suggest an analogy with depression brought on by negative life circumstances and manifested with physical complaints.

Amok. Found in Malaysia, the Philippines, and Thailand, the syndrome presents with a sudden clouding of consciousness with intense rage, reckless agitation, and homicidal aggression, frequently with a fatal outcome. As early as the 1770s, Captain Cook described in his log causeless terrible aggressions on the islands of the Malay Archipelago, and Stefan Zweig used the syndrome as a romantic metaphor in his novel that shares its name. Amok is preceded by seclusion, gloomy introspection, and autonomous signs of increasing tension, culminating in extreme excitation followed by total exhaustion and deep sleep. Not infrequently, the attacker is killed by his victims or commits suicide, or, in the case of survival, suffers from complete amnesia. The syndrome is sometimes regarded as a form of deliberate suicide through challenging the aggression of others in a community where strong taboos hang over the act of direct suicide. It is found only in men and, for this reason, a possible connection with the role of a man's honor in the tribe is suggested, but there are infectious factors to consider, as well.

Ataque de nervios. This state has been documented in Latin America and in large metropolitan areas of North America with a significant number of Latino immigrants. Its characteristic signs are sudden attacks of shaking, shouting, crying, tightness and heat in the chest and in the head, burning or prickling of the extremities, dizziness, and loss of memory. Local interpretations include possession by an evil spirit, thus making possible parallels with possession states to be drawn (Chapter 7); however, these patients rarely experience possession during such fits. Possession is posited as a secondary, post-hoc explanation, and their treatment is carried out through public rituals involving the support of others along with Catholic and indigenous symbols. These attacks are common during funerals, separations, divorces, and accidents. The similarity to panic attacks is obvious, but the psychogenic provocation, narrowed consciousness, and psychogenic improvement with the help of rituals also serve to illustrate the role of dissociation.

Susto. It exists in some communities of Latin America, particularly among the indigenous people of the Andes, and includes various symptoms that all share a "loss of spirit" as their supposed primary cause: anxiety, insomnia, loss of appetite, diarrhea, vomiting, sweating, fear, and oppression. The syndrome is usually either subsequent to some traumatic incident leading to the "detachment" of the patient's spirit from the body, or connected with processing some trauma from the past. The cultural version is, again, a post-hoc explanation and implies treatment with rituals of support, sweating, massage, and diet. The same clinical picture also manifests in some pre-menstrual syndromes in these communities.

Taijin kyofusho. This syndrome, widespread in Japan, includes experiencing intolerable shame at one's own appearance, body parts, or odor from different organs which might have a repulsive effect on others. Unlike the "European" sensitive reference idea (either delusional or overvalued), where other people show peculiar attitudes which are inexplicable to the individual, and, for this reason, become inserted into paranoid subject matter, in taijin kyofusho the individual is the source of unpleasant signals to others, causing their repulsion. The syndrome symbolizes the inherently Eastern emotion of shame from the possibility of offending others, as well as submission to the community, *le bon ton*, and rituals. It usually leads to home seclusion and total isolation in order to prevent any potential public insult. Although it has been interpreted as the Japanese version of social phobia, there is a certain distinction—the sociophobe is consumed by the fear of being embarrassed in the presence of others, while the person with taijin kyofusho is convinced that he or she causes disgust towards himself or herself due to appearance. When this conviction is absolute, the syndrome is a delusional disorder. The non-delusional variant is relatively common in the general population, among those with traumatic and harsh childhoods, the introverted, the extremely shy, or individuals with a predisposition to real physical or autonomous peculiarities, such as easy blushing.

Sinbyong. In Korea, affected women are regarded as shamans who are chosen by spirits. The syndrome's manifestations, such as excitement, hearing voices, and abundant autonomous symptoms, are considered morbid ("illness of the soul"), yet are also believed to be caused by the spirits to signify being summoned. The role of the shaman in Korean culture is an ambivalent one, and therefore women frequently refuse to accept the call of the spirits; the relatives of those who do accept it are ashamed of them. By accepting the call, they deny their own sexuality, replacing it with the ecstasy of the shaman ritual. A shamanic summoning of women may be interpreted as compensation for their traditionally limited scope of contribution outside the home. After either accepting the shaman's role or rejecting it, they calm down and the syndrome's manifestations disappear.

Windigo. A folk myth belonging to the Algonquians of Canada, it refers to a huge monster (wendigo or wihtiko—a giant) inhabiting the forests, attacking and eating people, but sparing the lives of children as it waits for them to grow up and gain weight. It has the power to transform adults, children, and animals into cannibals. This syndrome encompasses the fear of turning into a cannibal, conviction that this has already happened, real cannibalism, or suicidal behavior as a way to escape cannibalism.

Latah. It exists in Southeast Asia, mainly in Malaysia and on Java in Indonesia, and is only found in women. It presents with an acute reaction, sometimes during ceremonies (like weddings), intended to scare others with dramatic and scattered motor behavior, chaotic or stereotype movements, yelling, scanning, echolalia, or sudden acts of aggression using simple tools such as knives, boiled water, hot cooking oil, or stones. It is more prevalent among marginalized and poor people, or those who have lost their status in the community.

Zar. The word represents both the spirit that possesses people and various techniques for its neutralization or conciliation. It has ancient origins in Ethiopia, and in the 19th century was transferred to Egypt, acquiring a Sufi pattern under Islamic influence. Like most African spirits (Chapter 7), Zar inhabits a parallel invisible reality. It is also prone to expressing caprice and irritability towards some of the host's actions, and then the reproached one performs a series of rituals to calm the spirit. Besides its normative version, the cult has further analogues which are severely abnormal, such as psychoses among Ethiopian immigrants in Israel with altered states of consciousness, total possession by Zar, mutism, inarticulate speech, and involuntary movements.

Whakama. A behavioral model found in the Maori of New Zealand and in other parts of Polynesia, it includes acknowledging a lower status, submission, humility, and manifestations of shame, doubt, inadequacy, and seclusion. It is usually a sign of some real failure, loss of honor, or committed sin. This behavior, which can affect individuals or groups, is not considered pathological, and help is sought out only in extreme cases. An analogy with depression is far from certain, especially when the manifestation is collective and displays aggression.

Avanga. A traditional belief in Tonga culture, present in the South Pacific between the islands of Samoa and Fiji, about the role ancestral spirits play in the course of illness. It is a local variant of beliefs in spirit possession which are widespread in most cults and folk cosmogonies (Chapter 7). Those affected, usually women, believe that a spirit of some deceased relative is embodied in them and frequently shout, speak to the deceased, or visit the graveyards. Tonga culture has a complex system of denominations and concepts about the causes of disease, death, and misfortune, as well as their treatment or neutralization, which involve spirits, animals, (e.g., lizards), objects, and symbols.

Qigong. A holistic Chinese system for the coordination of bodily movements, breathing, and meditation, its aim is to improve one's health and reach a higher level of spirituality. It requires the cultivation of vital energy (qi—vital energy) and has deep roots in Confucianism, Daoism, Buddhism, and the traditions of Chinese medicine, meditation, and martial arts. Practiced in different forms as a means of esoteric teaching, it is persecuted in China; it was banned during the Cultural Revolution of the 1960s and 70s. In recent decades, it has gained popularity in many countries outside of China, being further developed into new concepts for therapy and self-improvement (like mindfulness). Over-participation in trance-like practices from traditional healing could cause induced states, resembling psychosis or self-absorption. Falun Gong, a variety of qigong with a more moralistic ideological platform, is currently being persecuted in China as a sect, and is often used as an occasion for political scandals and protests, while its followers are frequently involuntarily detained in psychiatric hospitals. Extreme engagement in the rituals and moralistic doctrine of Falun Gong could lead to anxiety, physical discomfort, agitation, weeping, and odd or aggressive behavior.

Koro. This encompasses a belief in Southeast Asia that the penis will shrink and retract into the abdominal cavity, accompanied by a feeling of horror. The afflicted will grasp the penis, also asking relatives to hold onto it, sometimes for days. The symbolic meaning of koro is related to the role of potency and paternal authority in these cultures. Analogies can be traced back to the ancient notion about sperm being essential to both health and life, as well as to the belief that each ejaculation causes the loss of vital strength, with death drawing closer. The fear of breast shrinkage and retraction is the female variant of koro.

Dhat. This is a belief in Southeast Asia, predominantly on the Indian subcontinent, that sperm is lost during urination. Like koro, it is associated with the role of sperm as a vital fluid in Hindu philosophy, and is accompanied by sexual disturbances such as premature ejaculation and erectile dysfunction, insomnia, low mood, and feelings of shame about masturbation. It is most commonly regarded as a variation of neurotic disorder with hypochondriac, and sometimes obsessive, concerns.

Tabanka. This syndrome, indigenous to Guinea-Bissau, is the inability to get over a separation combined with feelings of loss and grief. It looks like depression, but is limited to the specific experience of the breakup of a relationship. The word is of African or Creole origin, and also refers to a genre of Creole music.

Voodoo death. Beliefs in magic, and in its close relationship to health, illness, and fate are culturally universal (Chapters 6 and 7). What is specific to voodoo in the Caribbean and Polynesia (and among immigrants from there) is the power of curses cast by the voodoo magician, which may cause severe disease, misfortune, or death. Describing iatrogeny, Schipkowensky makes a psychological and physiological analysis of the mechanism behind voodoo death,[183] and also of the singular means of preventing it, contra-magic. A unique pathoanatomic protocol by Johns Hopkins Medical School from 1967[142] described the case of a young woman admitted shortly before her 23rd birthday with tachycardia, chest pain, shortage of breath, and syncope lasting almost a month. A careful medical examination did not uncover any pathology, while the patient shared with horror that she had been cursed at birth to die before she reached the age of 23. The day before her birthday, she died in the hospital.

There are plenty more culture specific idioms for the expression of distress, such as complaints of chest discomfort, overheating, and exhaustion resembling depression or cardio-vascular disease among the Sikhs of Punjab, or the brief yet intense rage states found in the Hopi of North America. In Japan, a new culture specific syndrome, *hikikimori* ("withdrawal into oneself"), has been described recently—a serious social and health problem, it affects approximately 1 million youth between 15 and 25 years of age. They do not leave their homes for years, often locking themselves in their rooms, only going out for food in the evening, severing all contact with relatives and friends, sleeping throughout the day, and surfing the Internet or reading manga (Japanese comics) at night. Besides opportunities for remote jobs online, or materializing one's social life on the web or via technology, other causes for the phenomenon include shame, introversion, emotional dependence on the mother, and the import of American culture, imposing extroversion onto even those for whom it is mentally alien.

Cultures, just like individuals from the same diagnostic category, do differ. Despite these differences, however, the characteristics they hold in common allow for the variegated faces of the phenomena to be settled into wider entities such as: amok in acute psychoses; susto and latah—in reactive states with dissociative pattern; or tabanka—in dysthymia. This categorization is convenient because it spares cognitive efforts. It is, however, debatable from an anthropological position due to its evident negligence of these syndromes' social construction according to the local cosmogony. Encountering what is culturally unknown carries two opposing risks: overpathologization or underestimation of pathology. All individual pathologies, not just the rare, exotic ones, are manifested within a certain context, for instance, when the patient and psychiatrist come from different social layers yet share a common culture. Individual idiosyncrasies must be accounted for on a biological level because we are also biologically unique. For this reason, culturally-sensitive psychiatric practices begin not abroad, but at home.

12 Treatment and Culture

> A strange disease requires a strange cure.
>
> W. Shakespeare

Beyond the technological framework of medicine, the expectations and means of health care delivery are definitely influenced by cultural attitudes. Health care transformations are more visible and understandable on the political and economic levels. The main change is, however, cultural, and can be briefly defined as a transition from paternalism to autonomy.[154] This transition modifies traditionally undisputed roles. The physician is no longer the savior from A.J. Cronin's novels who travels with his leather bag through snowdrifts to a woman in labor, nor is he an undisputed authority, but this new physician is an expert offering therapeutic services. Patients are not the passive recipients of prescriptions, but rather are informed customers who may accept or refuse these services. The degree to which a patient's choice is assisted in his best interest by a doctor determines a model of either partnership—with a high degree of such assistance—or one of consumerism, wherein services are offered like any other commodity with advertising, competition, and the ultimate aim of being sold. A contradiction of the health care context in societies going through a state of transition exists between the "liberal" consumerist model of service delivery and "conservative" paternalistic mentalities in attitudes held towards the patient.

The central place of patient autonomy and informed consent in bioethics[32, 179] has been determined by changes within a broader cultural context in which the role of one's inner experience and inter-subjectivity continues to grow. This context is characterized by the permeable border between object and subject, declining rigidity of roles, and new meaning being given to human identity, and even to the self in virtual reality.[209] The postmodern worldview is nuanced and allows for different viewpoints to redefine one and the same phenomenon. It features increased prevalence of the ecological over the ontological, of interpretation over perception, and—when it comes to research—of ethnographic and clinical observations over external measurements. The role of subjective experience is growing compared to more "objective" descriptions[139, 157] and this is true not only for aesthetics, but also science and health care. The convenient, singularly correct point of view is no longer present, while firm concepts get deconstructed into sets of views about them. In this context, the doctor-patient relationship is one between two subjects, not between a subject and an object—a relationship built on dialog, not obedience.

These changes and ethical rules are not universal. On the contrary, autonomy and informed consent are the achievements of individualistic cultures. For many traditional cultures with a preponderance of collective values, these measures are difficult to apply.[32] The very idea of asking a mentally ill person whether he wants to be treated would be ridiculed in many communities; the extent to which this happens is a clear sign of the culture's influence.[13,154] Coercion in psychiatry is in direct antagonism with autonomy. A large empirical study on coercive treatment measures in 10 European countries[56, 154] has illustrated the roles played by service, cultural, and inter-subjective factors, as well as how they affect clinical outcomes. Like other countries in Southern and Eastern Europe, and unlike the Northern or Western European participants in this project, Bulgaria's share of informal and covert coercion is much higher than legally applied coercion. The cultural roots of informal coercion in this country are both old[29, 154] and illustrative of culture's domination over legal norms—or of unwritten over written rules. Perceptions of coercion are high, both in voluntarily and involuntarily hospitalized patients: for two thirds of them, their perception remains high even after hospital discharge, and regardless of clinical improvement. Covert coercion, especially in emergency admissions, is associated with poorer clinical and social indicators, as well as reduced compliance to treatment after discharge, as compared to legally involuntary patients. It turns out that out of all the numerous clinical and demographic variables contained in the "black box" of hospital treatment, its medium-term outcome is best predicted by levels of functioning and satisfaction due to treatment in the first week following admission, and by the absence of an emergency hospitalization.[154]

Attempting to delve deeper into the organizational culture of medical institutions may throw light on the contradiction between autonomy and the mentality of traditional medicine, thus making it more intelligible. Hospitals are relatively stiff and closed institutions, with their own symbols, hierarchy, jargon, folklore, and secrets. A stay in hospital imposes the loss of many markers of identity. Attempts to break apart the secrets and internal rules result in group anxiety and mobilization of group defenses. As with other guild cultures, these defenses are institutionalized and acquire the status of regulated behaviors.

If we assess the organization of hospitals according Hofstede's dimensions, for the masculinity/femininity dimension it can be specified as masculine (although women prevail in hospital teams) because of values like ambitiousness, persistence, competitiveness, and diligence. For the uncertainty avoidance dimension, the abundance of stress, impatience, tension, bans, excessive control, rigorous observance of rules and boundaries, and suspicions towards divergence all create a high level of uncertainty in hospitals' organization. In the power distance index, external markers of status such as titles, parking places, offices, and the distance between superiors and subordinates define it as a culture with a high power distance. On the individualism/collectivism spectrum, the priority of collective values leaves no doubt about the predominantly collective orientation of hospitals' organization, while for the short term/long term orientation dimension, the domination of current and immediate interests and planning places it closer to the short-term pole.

The signs of these characteristics are a strict hierarchy, resistance to change, reproducibility of the rules, the clear demarcation between those inside the culture and others, suspiciousness towards control and publicity, and high levels of technologization and care, with a relative tendency to neglect the inner experience of illness. To some extent, these traits explain patients' search for alternative treatments.

Another characteristic of the contemporary mental healthcare context is the increasing occurrence of over-diagnosis—diagnosing diseases in spite of their absence, or assigning a more severe diagnosis in the presence of a milder disease. It is a general trend in medicine and is not specific to psychiatry alone. Reasons behind it have risen with the development of science and new treatments, along with cultural factors. The endophenotypes that are common for both healthy and unwell individuals confirm the dimensional transition between norm and pathology, and establish an argument which supports focusing on clinically insignificant signs. The discovery of new treatments for physiological manifestations, for instance nevus or stress, validate these manifestations as pathological. Over-diagnosis also runs parallel to the cultural fashion of health fads among the wealthy who share an obsession with healthy food, exercise, and a quest for immortality (e.g., freezing stem cells), and has drawn some medical disciplines in closer to the cosmetic industry. The competitive traits of developed countries, along with perfectionist expectations, depreciate anything that does not meet those lofty goals, and there is a tendency towards pathologization to the extent that having good health becomes identified as achieving perfection. In psychiatry, such a connection echoes the moralistic views about mental illness from the 19th century. Thus, notions of normalcy are narrowed, and human diversity becomes flatter while psychopathology is trivialized.

One of the main manifestations of over-diagnosis in psychiatry is found in the expansion of the bipolar spectrum—it has replaced and is similar to the expansion of the schizophrenia spectrum some decades ago. The spectrum's expansion embraces daily variations of bipolarity, undistinguishable from temperament, and reciprocally restricts the scope of unipolar depression with the tendency to erase it as a diagnosis. Only 43 % of patients with bipolar affective disorder (BAD) meet the criteria for this diagnosis when interviewed in a structured way,[226] and among children and adolescents in the USA this diagnosis has increased forty times in the last 40 years.[49] Furthermore, diagnoses of attention deficit with hyperactivity disorder (ADHD) have risen sixteen-fold over the last 20 years in the USA.[86]

Over-diagnosis is also manifested in the pathologization of aging. The cultural cult worshiping youth, health, and sex appeal neglects other qualities, frequently summarized as wisdom, which have been the reasoning behind the special status held by the elderly in traditional communities for millennia. With a harmonious transition through the preceding life cycle phases, old age reaches a level of integrity and capacity for existential understanding, illustrated by Leo Tolstoy in *The Death of Ivan Ilyich* as "the insight that when he had walked upwards, he had in fact been going downwards, and that when he had thought he was going downwards, he had in fact lived a full life". Contemporary studies show that the quality of life in elderly people suffering from physical illness is higher than in adults with the same afflictions.[111] In old age, personality pathologies, schizophrenia, affective disorders, obsessive-compulsive disorder, addictions, and aggressive tendencies improve—yet this comes at the price of increased dementia risk. Another manifestation of over-diagnosis is the lowering of diagnostic thresholds, made official with the introduction of the DSM-5 in the USA with its inclusion of many sub-thresholds and non-pathological signs within the categories. Five decades before this current trend, Schipkowensky (Fig. 16) emphatically declared, "The most common disease is the *diagnosis*".[183]

The frequency of singular psychiatric symptoms in the general population is indeed high: around 50 % of all people have experienced at least one phobia during their life, 50 % have had at least one panic attack, and around 5 % have heard a voice.[59] Single instances of symptoms, however, are not evidence of underlying syndromes or diseases. A single increase in blood pressure does not indicate hypertension, nor does a single panic attack mean that one has a panic disorder. The expansion of diagnostics based on the descriptive aspect of symptoms does not account for the essential features of psychopathology (Chapter 4): its quantitative distinction from the norm and the deterioration of functioning. There is no epidemic of mental disorders (as suggested in popularized, sensational terms); rather, there is an epidemic of labels being assigned to sub-threshold manifestations.

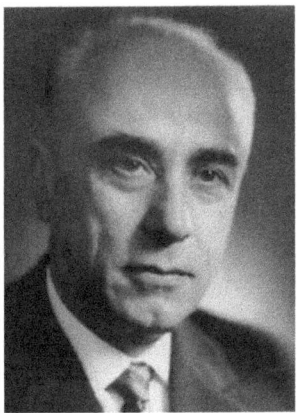

Fig. 16: Nikola Schipkowensky (1906–1976)

One major consequence of over-diagnosis is the blurred boundary between norm and pathology, which includes the invasion of diagnostic labels into the territory of health. This boundary is a relative one, and obscuring it further only leads to relativism in the definition of psychiatry itself and paradigmatic helplessness. With such obsessing over health, a diagnosis allows for abuse to be exerted with expert power. A product of this abuse is *the shadow of diagnosis*: once pronounced, all of one's problems in life are attributed to the diagnosis. This is a convenient—and, for this reason, steadily reproduced—explanatory model for relatives, doctors, law enforcement agencies, and others. The extension of psychiatry into the territory of health reduces psychopathology to daily experience and obligingly offers arguments to antipsychiatry.

Another consequence of over-diagnosis is over-treatment: the former leads to the latter (and is not infrequently done with this intention). Over-treatment causes a paradoxical situation—excessive treatment of mild conditions where it is *not necessary*, and insufficient treatment where it is *essential*. Psychiatry deserts more severe pathologies at the expense of milder ones. People with chronic schizophrenia remain inadequately cared for, while people with minimal anxiety or affective symptoms are provided lavish amounts of medications and enjoy frequent visits, particularly when they are in good social and economic standing. Thereby, psychiatry betrays its fundamental mission—to help the *severely* mentally ill. Historically, it has never dealt with milder or more common pathologies,[35] and this continues to be the case in most of the world.

The treatment of minimal clinical manifestations leads to erroneous conclusions regarding treatment. Analogous to type 1 or type 2 statistical errors, determining the presence or absence of some significant difference when precisely the opposite is evident, similar false conclusions can be deducted from treating sub-threshold or absent symptoms. If a transitional or grief reaction is spontaneously surmounted, a conclusion may be drawn that the treatment works—when there has actually been a natural return to the norm (type 1 erroneous conclusion)—or, on the other hand, the remittance of minimal or absent symptoms can lead to the conclusion that the treatment has not worked (type 2 error) even though it is, in fact, effective, yet the chance to demonstrate its effectiveness has not been forthcoming in the absence of pathology. Other consequences of the premature treatment of minimal clinical manifestations are associated with the refusal of centuries-long effective practices, such as watchful observation.

Among the cultural consequences of over-diagnosis is medicalizing normal human experiences, such as sadness, distractedness, joy, and rage. Human nature and life events are given medical explanations; problems and failures—diagnoses. The diversity of human life is reduced to a peculiar "living by quotes" (T. Mann): as in the great monotheistic doctrines where each human situation finds an explanation behind it in the Holy Scripture, so too, in modern psychiatry is each constellation of human experiences and behaviors threatened by diagnosis. The search for medical solutions stands in the way of achieving solutions through other means, and hence, mass over-diagnoses offer a medical alibi to human problems inherent to simply existing, depriving people of the opportunity to actually cope with them. For instance, the attribution of poor school performance to ADHD when it is absent deprives pupils, parents, and teachers of opportunities to cope with the real causes. The main bioethical consequence of over-diagnosis is the erosion of physician integrity and—its obvious result—the unnecessary treatment of healthy people.

The role of cultural contexts for treatment is diverse. Psychotherapy, for example, is considered to be a culturally specific approach[208] which is hardly applicable, or inefficient, in non-Western populations. Psychotherapy is indeed an undoubtedly cultural product. The search for hidden meaning in the words of the Talmud resembles the psychoanalytic method, bringing psychoanalysis closer to Jewish mysticism. Cognitive-behavioral therapy, on the other side, is a culturally adapted version of the modern rational view of life in developed countries. Schipkowensky's "healing silence"[183] suggests analogies with the practices of Hesychasm (from the Greek, meaning to keep silence), a mystical tradition in the Eastern Orthodox Church that was widespread in the medieval Balkans, as

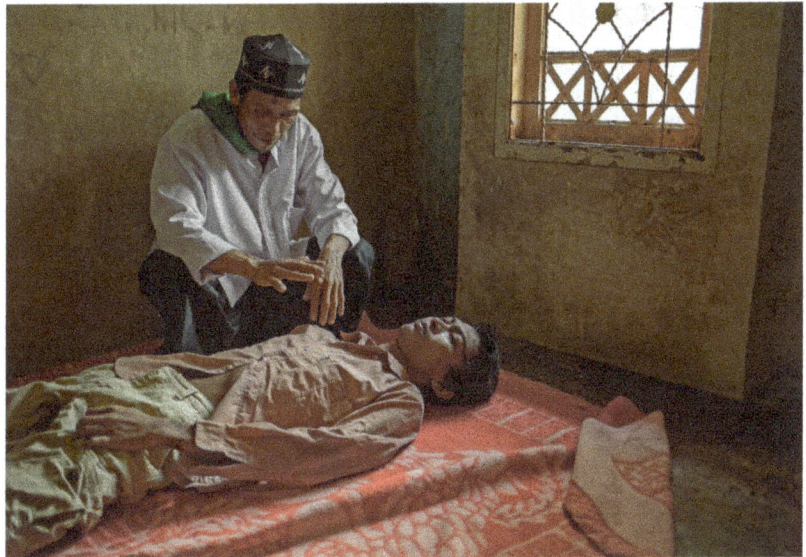

Fig. 17: A traditional healing session, Indonesia (Courtesy to A. S. Reese)

well as with regional attitudes held up to this day which expect problems to be resolved without speaking about them. The search for intrapsychic causes of suffering is rooted in the concept of personal responsibility in the Judeo-Christian world, and is alien to traditional communities.

With folk treatments (Fig. 17), the healer treats the subjective perception of illness, and not the disease, in a biomedical sense. In conventional medicine, the doctor treats the disease, but not the subjective perception of illness. The use of ritual objects such as amulets may have direct physical and instrumental effects, but also symbolic ones, corresponding to the cultural need for dependence and somatization. A charismatic alliance with the healer, along with a sense of coherence with cultural meanings, clarity, perception, and predictability, is the basis for therapeutic efficiency. Alcoholism in some Native Americans is treated with group tribal rituals; the fear of semen loss in India is treated with dhat; yoga and other rituals return the "lost" souls of the mentally ill in Nepal; and rituals of exorcism, releasing the afflicted from possession or magic, are so widely accepted in Indonesia that they are practiced in state psychiatric hospitals.[142, 145, 208] Magical cures belong to a common narrative within the varied stories corresponding to magical explanations: exorcising spirits when possessed by them, neutralizing negative energy fields, casting spells with evil eyes, undoing magic with bewitching, fasting with intoxication, infusions with metabolic disturbance, extra-sensory influences, being zombified by paranormal forces, etc. The ancient principle of like curing like (*similia similibus curantur*) is adhered to strictly.

Seeking help for mental disorders can be hindered or eased by many cultural barriers and bridges. Some minority or marginalized groups rarely seek the help of mental health services due to fears of stigma, suspiciousness, or mistrust. In traditional communities, help is sought out, as a rule, firstly from insiders, e.g., the extended family, local religious leaders and authorities, or the larger community. Being admitted into a psychiatric hospital is especially risky for Arab women because it either reduces their chances for marriage or increases the likelihood of divorce.[4] A competent approach to authentic community mental healthcare requires interaction between professionals and religious organizations or informal local leaders in order to inform them about available mental health services, facilitate referrals, preventatively discuss ungrounded fears and prejudices, and integrate cultural and religious values into the delivery of care. Subcultures with supernatural beliefs and traditions can usually clearly distinguish between trances and talking to spirits as acceptable practices or as signs of illness;[146] symptoms of psychosis are perceived as morbid everywhere (Chapters 6 and 7).[134, 135, 172] For this reason, interacting with the local healers (instead of opposing them) is not only feasible, but also fruitful. In East Africa I have witnessed a curious working guild agreement with the watchawi traditional healers: magic treatments for neurotic symptoms, and referral to psychiatrist in cases of psychosis or seizures.

Cultural sensitivity in treatment delivery requires knowledge of the specific role models, attitudes, sources of support and motivation for treatment, and capacity to account for cultural transfer and contra transfer[208] in the mutual adjustment of mentalities and expectations, as well as to enhance compliance. The intake of drugs also has its cultural nuances like symbolism, form, taste, and importance to the diet. During Ramadan, it is possible to prescribe Muslims long-acting medications, taken once daily after sunset or before sunrise, and in severe conditions the religious obligation to fast can be acceptably postponed. There are also ethnic and racial differences in drug assimilation due to differences in the P450 cytochrome, some enzymes, or in food.

According to Socrates, Ancient Greek physicians could not successfully treat most diseases because they had incomplete notions about the body's wholeness, erroneously targeting their efforts to its parts, while the good health of the whole was a precondition for the wellbeing of the parts.[183] And Avicenna divided all diseases into three groups, calling one of them diseases of the temperament, and including in it practically all mental and internal disorders.[14] The holistic approach towards illness and the psychosomatic deduction of physical diseases from temperament, though they represent traditions going back millennia, were substituted by contemporary medicine—autistic in its way of thinking, according to Bleuler—with technological advances on local micro-levels, but still failing to integrate them in toto. This is the paradox of the history of medicine: when physicians were almost helpless, they were believed unconditionally, but now with the much higher efficiency of modern healthcare, the personal touch has been lost and trust eroded.[148] Alternative treatments are sought mostly for the holisticity that they offer. Besides magical rituals, they include spiritual practices, meditation, naikan—a specific mobilizing method of self-interrogation and self-castigation in Japan[208]—new age treatments, and others. Spirituality is an antidote to narcissism and the experience of being in a vacuum. The integration of spiritual elements into a complex therapy is not in conflict with taking medication or with personal beliefs, and has shown its efficacy in the philosophy of the twelve-step approach in the treatment of addiction and severe personality pathologies, as well as other therapeutic programs. Unlike cultural differences, spirituality is focused on what people hold basically in common, summed up by V. Frankle with the statement that there is no human being who can say that he has never failed, does not suffer, or will not die.[61]

The role of the psychiatrist also has its cultural limitations, and has been the subject of redefinition across different contexts. Psychiatry assimilates theories and practices from both biological and humanitarian disciplines, and a psychiatrist communicates with different realities, switching over like an experienced interpreter between their means of expression: health and illness, fantasy and reality, biochemical and psychological correlates, complaints and symbols, process and content, self-reflection and empathy. The Renaissance spirit-body dualism is merely a minor burden, compared to the multilateral context of the contemporary "alienist" practice—with its increasing cultural fluidity, dilution of meanings, and the accelerating velocity of changes in context and in manifestations of psychopathology. Parallel to the development and introduction of new therapies, the chronic presence and cost of illnesses increase.[152] Social control does not allow for the personalization of care outside limiting standards and algorithms, and the increasing social pressure on professional loyalty causes a conflict of duty, imposing the role of double agent onto the psychiatrist: one who serves both the patient's and society's interests. In such a milieu, the appeal to compassion from Maimonides' prayer for the physician seems to be also culture specific.

13 Epilogue: After Tomorrow

> The answer is blowing in the wind.
>
> *B. Dylan*

In the epilogue of his book *Zen and the Art of Motorcycle Maintenance*, R. Pirsig makes a brilliant comparison between the Renaissance era and the modern age with the eloquent reminder that Renaissance period was only defined as such years later.[160] Unlike the evaluation of later generations, its contemporaries had extremely negative opinions about their time. The journeys which led to great geographical discoveries were perceived as simple adventures; new dramatic works, poetry, and paintings—as in poor taste; and the urban way of life—a moral disgrace. The era's scientific discoveries and social upheavals were met with shock and were viewed as signs of an overt rejection of Medieval rules, security, and predictability. The indecency of stage plays (frequently welcomed by throwing rotten eggs), widespread drunkenness in ports, on the streets, and at universities, undisguised prostitution, and widespread disrespect to social norms, traditions, and even the church left no doubt about the collapse of revered centuries-old feudal values. These changes were experienced painfully. The reference term "Renaissance", as well as the evaluation of progress made in all areas of life, would only appear almost two centuries later.

Similarly, today's cultural changes are perceived with nostalgia for old values and without recognizing their potential for the future. The velocity of these changes is scary, leaving many to feel that global chaos is replacing the coziness and slower pace from the hierarchically more ordered past. The spirit of negation, peculiar to cultures in transition, sees only the darker side of things, makes fatalistic prognoses, and demonizes everything associated with change: the Internet, drugs, "today's youth", violence, lechery, terrorism, democracy, free movement of immigrants, or whatever other vice, depending on the underlying ideologemes, scale of fear, and lack of personal liberty. Again, as in centuries past, the huge *potential for development* in troubled times—eloquently illustrated by descriptions of the epoch which would be later called the Renaissance and by the astonishing insights of Toynbee[207] about the spiritually motivating power of human history—goes unrecognized. Such troubled times are the *bouillon primordial* for the rise of new civilizations.

And psychopathology is the price that mankind pays for this—the price of its own uneasiness, curiosity, and quest-seeking. The alternative is security. For this reason, when human development accelerates, collective anxiety increases (and so do anxiety disorders). Cultures with more predictable and secure lifestyles are sedated, do not offer any stimulus for change, and lack the potential for development. Psychopathology is less prevalent there and, clinically, is frozen. In troubled times, psychopathology grows more prevalent and clinically dynamic. The dramatized experience of transience is, to a certain extent, inevitable: the tempo with which cultural sedation and security are broken is such that it offers no pause to make sense of what is going on. Signs of revival will be discovered later, but not while the change is happening. Because the skill of looking ahead is not innate to those "vaunting the past" (*laudatores temporis acti*)[51] or to "grey reverents"[94] with their constricted, dark, fearful, and nostalgic thinking, it is precisely such thinking which feeds into the medium of insecurity and post-truth. To employ Eco's metaphor for visionary effects, the dwarfs should step on the giants' shoulders.

Evolution is gaining speed. Millions of years were needed for the hunter-gatherer to begin to speak and recognize his own experiences; millennia passed before the horse's domestication or the creation of the wheel and monotheistic religions; and it took centuries for scientific and technological progress, industrialization, and the development of modern healthcare. Yet it has only taken decades for the rise of the Internet, digital technologies, new information units such as the meme,[23] and even new identities. History compresses time, and the temporal dimension accelerates. The cultural consequences of this are difficult to grasp. In a sense, culture enters a kind of contradiction with itself because its purpose is to preserve meanings and experiences, transmitting them through generations rather than altering them rapidly.

Virtual reality has created a kingdom of ideas above the biosphere in which *memes* (from memory) multiply and acquire their own existence as memotypes, via analogy with genotypes. The Buddhist appeal for liberation from the belongings of one's thoughts has been technologically fulfilled by the collective storage of thoughts, thus leading to what is sometimes called augmented humanity. Language, as a catalyst of culture, is also changing, deserting entire linguistic layers and being enriched with new jargons such as technobabble. Along with these changes, however, the semantic landscape is blurred by the post-truth confusion of facts and values and by the euphemisms of politically correct speech, in this way replacing the traditional, commonsense ecology of fear with a new ecology of disguise. Classical individual identities are transformed into something more fluid, with loose boundaries, closer to collective affiliations[202, 209] and with vague localization—this is why it is possible for new forms of identity disturbances to appear in psychopathology. These changes in identity are similar to some dissociative phenomena and, in a sense, turn the individual self back into its pre-historical collective prototype.

The ideological and scientific revolutions have undermined the human sense of uniqueness.[139] Copernicus demonstrated that man is not at the center of the universe; Darwin—that he has no divine origin but is nearer to animals than was previously supposed; and Freud—that he is not aware of his motives and is irrational. The fourth paradigmatic turn, associated now with digital technologies and artificial intelligence, shows that man is not unique in his capacity to think, either. The psyche itself is no longer interpreted as being fixed in objective reality, but rather as a changeable social construct which is subject to constant revision and influence by cultural dominants.

The study of genetics is contributing to a personalized medicine of the future, presumably with individual genome-specific treatment, but it is not going to solve the problem of mental illnesses and their etiology. The neurosciences may enter into the most intimate mechanisms of engrams processing and the relationship between genes, proteins, and neurophysiological activity, but they cannot embrace the connection between this activity and mental experience. The *human being*, and not the brain, is feeling and thinking for this reason.[183] The brain is an instrument that produces electric impulses and neuromediators; however, the connection between them and love or hate is a connection capable of deducing the immaterial from the material, which remains gnoseologically unachievable on the current stage of evolution. As we investigate animals and discover things that are not accessible to their cognition, so too will the great conundrums concerning the essence of the mind, and psychopathology as part of it, receive possible solutions from higher species, or from higher research paradigms that may outgrow the objective metric approach. Solutions to these problems may also arrive as products of other disciplines, such as physics, according to which information and experiences may be contained within quanta, or they may result from combinations of paradigms and disciplines, like this one suggested by Einstein: "Science without religion is crippled, and religion without science is blind".

As they have done until now throughout history, cultural changes will lead to changes in psychopathology and illness behavior. The frequency of schizophrenia will probably decrease, as evidenced by the evolutionary curve of its prevalence over time (Chapter 7). At the expense of this, the frequency of related disorders from the autistic spectrum will increase: from mild eccentricities to more severe developmental deviations with cognitive deficit and physical anomalies. Medical advances will make possible the survival of many carriers of congenital aberrations, and increasingly liberal attitudes towards them will lead to more couples choosing to preserve the fetus, even with plausible prenatal screening. Parallel to the decrease of schizophrenia, the portion of psychoses due to drug use will increase, besides, with clinical pictures that can be "prescribed" in advance and programmed by molecular design. The prevalence of depression will remain high, although it is possible that milder depressions will be terminologically and conceptually replaced by adaptation or stress reactions. The prevalence of anxiety disorders is functional to the velocity of cultural changes: increasing with great speed and decreasing with slow speed. The manifestation of anxiety will increasingly transform from its classical models to defensive behaviors, such as the Japanese hikikimori (Chapter 11). The portion of dementia patients will increase too, along with the role of instrumental assessment.

Rehabilitation, and not utopian radical treatments, will become the ultima ratio of mental healthcare, and will determine its pattern. It will improve, not due to effective treatment or as a result of humane concerns, but due to decreased stigma. An excess of eccentric othernesses in the real or virtual world will turn mental illness into a more banal and everyday experience, depriving it of enigma and prejudices. On the one hand, psychiatry will become trivialized, its halo of mystery removed as it transforms into an ordinary neuro-discipline, working with neuroimaging methods. On the other, the need for its eternal vocation of insight, understanding, and compassion—especially in the environment of digital identities and alienation—will increase.

List of Figures

Fig. 1:	Bulgarians, painting by Stoyan Venev	38
Fig. 2:	Karl Jaspers (1883–1969)	46
Fig. 3:	Kurt Schneider (1887–1967)	58
Fig. 4:	Emil Kraepelin (1856–1926), around the time of his voyage to Java, 1903	67
Fig. 5:	Sigmund Freud (1856–1939)	68
Fig. 6:	Symptom formation in psychopathology	71
Fig. 7:	An Arab Orthodox Coptic priest exorcises a Muslim compatriot	78
Fig. 8:	Hristo Petrov (1901–1944)	98
Fig. 9:	Emanuil Sharankov (1903–1997)	100
Fig. 10:	Granny Zlata from the village of Bulgari, the last genuine nestinar in the Strandzha mountains	101
Fig. 11:	Patients with catatonia, illustration from Kraepelin's textbook, 1899 edition	114
Fig. 12:	John Nash, Nobel prize winner in economics, diagnosed with schizophrenia	119
Fig. 13:	The Anatomy of Melancholy by R. Burton, 1628 edition	125
Fig. 14:	Deconstruction of the depressive syndrome	130
Fig. 15:	A rakiya still, the Bulgarian forum	137
Fig. 16:	Nikola Schipkowensky (1906–1976)	157
Fig. 17:	A traditional healing session, Indonesia	159

List of Tables

Tab. 1:	Basic distinctions between cultures	27
Tab. 2:	Axes for assessing a mentally ill person in the Roman tribunal, 1st century BCE	63
Tab. 3:	Basic differences in psychopathology between cultures	72
Tab. 4:	Results from the International Pilot Study of Schizophrenia (IPSS) in different cultures, follow up for 26 years	117
Tab. 5:	Results from the Determinants of Outcomes and Course of Severe Mental Disorders (DOSMED) in different cultures, follow up for 15 years	118
Tab. 6:	Results from the Reduction and Assessment of Psychiatric Disability (RAPyD) in different cultures, follow up over 14 to 16 years	119

References

1. Adityanjee M. D., Raju G. S. P., Khandelwal S. K. Current status of multiple personality disorder in India. *Am J Psychiatry* 1989; 146: 1607–1610
2. Ahmed S. H. Cultural influences on delusion. *Psychiatr Clin (Basel)* 1978; 11: 1–9
3. Alexander P. J., Joseph S., Das A. Limited utility of ICD-10 and DSM-IV classification of dissociative and conversion disorders in India. *Acta Psychiatr Scand* 1997; 95: 177–182
4. Al-Krenawi A., Graham, J. R. Culturally sensitive social work: practice with Arab clients in mental health settings. *Health & Social Work* 2000; 25: 9–22
5. Al-Subaie A., Alhamad A. Psychiatry in Saudi Arabia. In I. Al-Junün (ed.). *Mental illness in the Islamic world*. Madison: International Universities Press, 2000, 205–233
6. American Psychiatric Association. *Diagnostic and Statistical Manual of Mental Disorders, 5th ed. (DSM-5)*. Washington, DC: American Psychiatric Press, 2014
7. Andreasen N. C. Negative symptoms in schizophrenia. Definition and reliability. *Arch Gen Psychiatry* 1982; 39: 784–788
8. Andreasen N. C. *Scale for the Assessment of Negative Symptoms (SANS)*. Iowa City: University of Iowa, 1984
9. Andreasen N. A unitary model of schizophrenia: Bleuler's "fragmented phrene" as schizencephaly. *Arch Gen Psychiatry* 1999; 56: 781–787
10. Andreasen N. DSM and the death of phenomenology in America: an example of unintended consequences. *Schizophr Bull* 2007; 33: 108–112
11. Angst J. European long-term follow-up studies of schizophrenia. *Schizophr Bull* 1988; 14: 501–513
12. Arnaudov M. *Studia on Bulgarian rites and legends. Part I Nestinarstvo. Part II Summer customs and magics* (in Bulgarian). Sofia: Universitetska biblioteka, 1924
13. Babiker I. E., Thorne P. Do psychiatric patients know what is good for them? *J Royal Soc Medicine* 1993; 86: 28–30
14. Babinov L. *The Arab medicine* (in Bulgarian). Sofia: Medicina i fizkultura, 1980
15. Berdyaev N. *The meaning of history* (transl. by G. Reavey). London: G. Bles, 1936

16. Berdyaev N. *The origin of Russian communism* (transl. by R. M. French). London: G. Bles, 1937
17. Berganza C. E. Broadening the international base for the development of an integrated diagnostic system in psychiatry. *World Psychiatry* 2003; 2, 1: 38–40
18. Bergman I. *The magic lantern: an autobiography* (1987, transl. by J. Tate). Chicago: University of Chicago Press, 1988
19. Berne E. *Games people play: the psychology of human relationships*. Middlesex: Penguin Books, 1972: 132–135
20. Berrios G. E. *The history of mental symptoms: descriptive psychopathology since nineteenth century*. Cambridge: Cambridge University Press, 1996
21. Bhugra D., Bhui K. (eds.) *Textbook of cultural psychiatry*. Cambridge: Cambridge University Press, 2007
22. Bilu Y., Beit-Hallahmi B. Dybbuk – possession as a hysterical symptom: psychodynamic and socio-cultural factors. *Isr J Psychiatry Relat Sci* 1989; 26: 138–149
23. Blackmore S. *The men machine*. Oxford: Oxford University Press, 1999
24. Blanchard J. J., Cohen A. S. The structure of negative symptoms within schizophrenia: implications for assessment. *Schizophr Bull* 2006; 32: 238–245
25. Bleuler E. *Dementia praecox, or the group of schizophrenias* (Bleuler E., 1911, transl. by J. Zunkin). New York: International Universities Press, 1950
26. Bleuler M. *The schizophrenic disorders. Long-term patient and family studies* (transl. by S. M. Clemens). New Haven: Yale University Press, 1978
27. Bonnell V., Hunt L. (eds.). *Beyond the cultural turn*. Berkeley: University of California Press, 1999
28. Bose R. Psychiatry and the popular conception of possession among Bangladeshis in London. *Int J Soc Psychiatry* 1997; 43: 1–15
29. Boyadjiev B, Onchev G. Legal and cultural aspects of involuntary psychiatric treatment regulation in post-totalitarian milieu: the Bulgarian perspective. *Eur J Psychiatry* 2007; 21, 3: 179–188
30. Braam A. W., Beekman A. T., Deeg D. J., et al. Religiosity as a protective factor of depression in later life; results from a community survey in the Netherlands. *Acta Psychiatr Scand* 1997; 96: 199–205
31. Brewerton T. D. Hyperreligiosity in psychotic disorders. *J Nerv Ment Disord* 1994; 182: 302–304
32. Brody E. Patients' rights: a cultural challenge to Western psychiatry. *Am J Psychiatry* 1985; 142: 58–62

33. Camic P. M., Rhodes J. E., Yardlew L. (eds.). *Qualitative research in psychology: expanding perspectives in methodology and design*. Washington, DC: American Psychological Association, 2003
34. Campbell M., Sibeko G., Mall S., et al. The content of delusions in a sample of South African Xhosa people with schizophrenia. *BMC Psychiatry* 2017; 17: 41
35. Cannabih Y. *History of psychiatry* (in Russion, 1928, reprint). Moscow: CTR MGP VOS, 1994
36. Caroff S. N., Mann S. C., Francis A., Fricchione G. L. (eds.). *Catatonia: from psychopathology to neurobiology*. Arlington: American Psychiatric Publishing, 2004
37. Church A. T. Culture and personality: toward an integrated cultural trait psychology. *J Personality* 2000; 68: 651–703
38. Church A. T., Lonner W. J. The cross-cultural perspective in the study of personality: rationale and current research. *J Cross-Cult Psychol* 1998; 29: 32–62
39. Ciompi L. Catamnestic long-term study on the course of life and aging of schizophrenics. *Schizophr Bull* 1980; 5: 606–618
40. Cloninger C. R. A systematic method for clinical description and classification of personality variants. *Arch Gen Psychiatry* 1987; 44: 573–588
41. Cooper J. E., Kendell R. E., Gurlend B. J., et al. *Psychiatric diagnosis in New York and London*. London: Oxford University Press: 1972
42. Cradock N., Owen M. J. Rethinking psychosis: the disadvantages of a dichotomous classification now outweigh the advantages. *World Psychiatry* 2007; 6, 2: 20–27
43. Crapo R. H. *Cultural anthropology: understanding ourselves and others* (2nd ed.). Guilford: The Dushkin Publishing Group Inc., 1990
44. Crow T. J. Schizophrenia as the price that homo sapiens pays for language: a resolution of the central paradox in the origins of species. *Brain Res Brain Res Rev* 2000; 31: 118–129
45. Dahl A. A. Problems concerning the concept of reactive psychosis. *Psychopathology* 1987; 20: 79–86
46. Darwin C. *The expression of emotion in man and animals*. London: John Murray, 1972
47. Diamond J. *The world until yesterday: what can we learn from traditional societies?* New York: Viking Press, 2012
48. Dubertret C., Gorwood P. The French concept of "psychose hallucinatoire chronique" – a preliminary form of schizophrenia? The role of late-life

psychosis in the anticipation hypothesis of schizophrenia. *Dialogues in Clinical Neuroscience: New Perspectives in Chronic Psychoses* 2001; 3: 296-303

49. Duffy A. Does bipolar disorder exist in children? A selected review. *Can J Psychiatry* 2007; 52: 409-417
50. Dyer G. *War: the lethal custom.* New York: Carroll & Graff Publishers, 2005
51. Eco U. *A passo di gambero.* Milano: Bompiani, 2006
52. Eliade M. *Le myth de l'eternal retour (nouvelle édition revue et augmenteé).* Paris: Gallimard, 1969
53. Emsley R. A., Niehaus D. J., Mbanga N. I., et al. The factor structure for positive and negative symptoms in South African Xhosa patients with schizophrenia. *Schizophr Res* 2001; 47: 149-157
54. Ferracuti S., Sacco R., Lazzari R. Dissociative trance disorder: clinical and Rorschach findings in ten persons reporting demon possession and treated by exorcism. *J Pers Assess* 1996; 66: 525-539
55. Fink M., Taylor M. A. *Catatonia: a clinician's guide to diagnosis and treatment.* Cambridge: Cambridge University Press, 2003
56. Fiorillo A., Giacco D., De Rosa C., et al. Patient characteristics and symptoms associated with perceived coercion during hospital treatment. *Acta Psychiatr Scand* 2012; 125: 460-467
57. Fotev G. *The Bulgarian melancholy* (in Bulgarian). Sofia: East-West, 2010
58. Foucault M. *Histoire de la folie.* Paris: Plon, 1961
59. Frances A. *Saving normal: an insider's revolt against out-of-control psychiatric diagnosis, DSM-5, Big Pharma, and the medicalization of ordinary life.* New York: Harper Collins Publishers, 2013
60. Frankfurt H. G. *On bullshit.* Princeton: Princeton University Press, 2005
61. Frankl V. *Man's search for meaning. An introduction to logotherapy* (1946). Boston: Beacon Press, 2006
62. Freud S. *Introduction to psychoanalysis* (transl. by G. S. Hall). New York: Boni and Liveright, 1920
63. Fromm E. *Escape from freedom.* New York: Farrar & Rinehart, 1941
64. Fullford K. W. M., Smirnov A. Y. U., Snow E. Concepts of disease and the abuse of psychiatry in the USSR. *Br J Psychiatry* 1993; 162: 801-810
65. Gaines A. D. Culture-specific delusions. Sense and nonsense in cultural context. *Psychiatr Clin North Am* 1995; 18: 281-301
66. Galanter M. (ed.). *Cults and new religious movements: a report of the Committee on psychiatry and religion.* Washington: APA, 1989

67. Ganev K., Onchev G., Ivanov P. A 16-year follow-up study of schizophrenia and related disorders in Sofia, Bulgaria. *Acta Psychiatr Scand* 1998; 98: 200–207
68. Ganev K., Onchev G., Ivanov P. *Chapter 20. RAPyD: Sofia, Bulgaria.* In K. Hopper, G.Harrison, A. Janca, N. Sartorius (eds.). *Recovery from schizophrenia: an international perspective.* Oxford: Oxford University Press, 2007: 227–239
69. Gelder M. G. A core curriculum in psychiatry for medical students. *Curr Opin Psychiatry* 1998; 11, 5: 491–492
70. Gift T. E., Strauss J. S., Young Y. Hysterical psychosis: an empirical approach. *Am J Psychiatry* 1985; 142: 345–347
71. Goff D. C., Brotman A. W., Kindlon D., Waites M., Amico E. The delusion of possession in chronically psychotic patients. *J Nerv Ment Dis* 1991; 179: 567–571
72. Graves R. *I, Claudius.* London: Arthur Barker, 1934
73. Greenberg D. Mysticism and psychosis: the fate of Ben Zoma. *Br J Med Psychology* 1992; 65: 223–235
74. Grigorieff V. *Religions du mond entire.* Alleurt: Marabout, 1996
75. Grisaru N., Budowski D., Wirtzum E. Possession by the "Zar" among Ethiopian immigrants to Israel: psychopathology or culture-bound syndrome? *Psychopathology* 1997; 30: 223–233
76. Hadjiisky I. *Optimistic theory for our people* (in Bulgarian). Sofia: Bulgarski pisatel, 1974
77. Hale A. S., Punninti N. R. Exorcism-resistant ghost possession treated with clopenthixol. *Br J Psychiatry* 1994; 165: 386–388
78. Hamdi E., Amin Y., Abou-Saleh M. T. Problems in validating endogenous depression in the Arab culture by contemporary diagnostic criteria. *J Affect Dis* 1997; 44: 131–143
79. Hamilton N. G. A critical review of object relations theory. *Am J Psychiatry* 1989; 146: 1552–1560
80. Harding C. M., Brooks G. W., Ashikaga T., Strauss J. S., Breier A. The Vermont longitudinal study of persons with severe mental illness. 1. Methodology, study samples and status after 32 years later. *Am J Psychiatry* 1987; 144: 718–726
81. Hasin D. S., Stinson F. S., Oqburn E., Grant B. F. Prevalence, correlates, disability, and comorbidity of DSM-IV alcohol abuse and dependence in the United States: results from the National Epidemiologic Survey on Alcohol and Related Conditions. *Arch Gen Psychiatry* 2007; 64: 830–842

82. Hassim J., Wagner C. Considering the cultural context in psychopathology formulations. *S Afr J Psych* 2013; 19, 1: 4–10
83. Hedelson P. M. *Qualitative research for health programmes.* Geneva: WHO/MNH/PSF/94.3, 1994
84. Helman C. G. Limits of biomedical explanation. *Lancet* 1991; 337: 1080–1082
85. Heyerdahl T. *Early man and the ocean.* New York: Doubleday & Co, 1979
86. Hinshaw S. P., Scheffler R. M. *The ADHD explosion: myths, medication, money, and today's push for performance.* New York: Oxford University Press, 2014
87. Hofstede G. Cultures and organizations: software of the mind. Maidenhead: McGraw-Hill, 1991
88. Hopper K., Harrison G., Janca A., Sartorius N. (eds.). *Recovery from schizophrenia: an international perspective.* Oxford: Oxford University Press, 2007
89. Huber G., Gross G., Schuttler R. A. A long-term follow-up study of schizophrenia: psychiatric course of illness and prognosis. *Acta Psychiatr Scand* 1975; 52: 49–57
90. Huizinga J. *Homo ludens* (1949). New York: Routledge, 1998
91. Huntington S. *The clash of civilizations and the remaking of world order.* New York: Simon & Schuster, 1996
92. IGDA Workgroup, WPA. IGDA. 7: Standardised multi-axial diagnostic formulation. *Br J Psychiatry* 2003; 182 (suppl. 45): s52–s54
93. IGDA Workgroup, WPA. IGDA. 8: Idiographic (personalised) diagnostic formulation. *Br J Psychiatry* 2003; 182 (suppl. 45): s55–s57
94. Ignatow A. *Psychologie des Kommunismus.* München: Iohanes Bergmans Verlag, 1985
95. Iida J. The current situation in regard to the delusion of possession in Japan. *Jpn J Psychiatry & Neurol* 1989; 43: 19–27
96. Jablensky A. *Schizophrenia – nosological unity and cultural variety* (in Bulgarian). Sofia: Medicina i fizkultura, 1986
97. Jablensky A. The syndrome – an antidote to spurious comorbidity. *World Psychiatry* 2004; 3, 1: 24–25
98. Jablensky A. Worldwide burden of schizophrenia. In B. J. Sadock, V. A. Sadock, P. Ruiz (eds.) *Kaplan & Sadock's comprehensive textbook of psychiatry*, 9th ed. Philadelphia: Lippincot Willliams & Wilkins, 2009: 1451–1462

99. Jablensky A., Hugler H., von Cranach M., Kalinov K. Kraepelin revisited: a reassessment and statistical analysis of dementia praecox and manic-depressive insanity in 1908. *Psychol Medicine* 1993; 23: 843–858

100. Jablensky A., Sartorius N., Ernberg G., et al. *Schizophrenia: manifestations, incidence, and course in different countries: a World Health Organization 10-country study*. Psychol Medicine, suppl. 20 (monograph). Cambridge: Cambridge University Press, 1992

101. Jablensky A., Schwarz R., Tomov T. WHO collaborative study on impairments and disabilities associated with schizophrenia. *Acta Psychiatr Scand* 1980; 62 (suppl 285): 152–163

102. Jackson M. (ed.). *Things as they are: new directions in phenomenological anthropology*. Bloomington: Indiana University Press, 1996

103. James W. *The varieties of religious experience*. Cambridge: Harvard University Press, 1985

104. Jaspers K. *General psychopathology* (7th ed.) (transl. by J. Hoenig & M. W. Hamilton). Baltimore: John Hopkins University Press, 1997

105. Jenkins J., Barrett R. (eds.). *Schizophrenia, culture and subjectivity*. Cambridge: Cambridge University Press, 2004

106. Jilek W. G. Transcultural psychiatry, quo vadis? *Transcult Psychiatr Newsletter* 1998; 16: 1–10

107. Jilek W. G. The early history of cultural psychiatry. *World Cult Psychiatr Res Rev* 2014; 9, 1: 3–15

108. Judt T. *Postwar: a history of Europe since 1945*. New York: Random House, 2011

109. Jung K. G. *Archetypes and the collective unconsciousness*. New Jersey: Princeton University Press, 1969

110. Kahlbaum K. L. *Catatonia or tension insanity* (Kahlbaum, 1874, transl. by Y. Levij & T. Pridan). Baltimore: Johns Hopkins University Press, 1973

111. Karel M. J., Gatz M., Smyer M. Ageing and mental health in the decade ahead: what psychologists need to know. *Am Psychologist* 2012; 67: 184–198

112. Kernberg O. F. The structural diagnosis of borderline organization. In P. Hartocollis (ed.). *Borderline personality disorders: the concept, the syndrome, the patient*. New York: International University Press, 1977, 87–121

113. Kessler R. C., Angermeyer M., Anthony J. C., et al. Lifetime prevalence and age-of-onset distributions of mental disorders in the World Health

Organization's World Mental Health Survey Initiative. *World Psychiatry* 2007; 6: 168-176

114. Khan M. M. (transl.). *The translation of the meanings of Sahîh Al-Bukhâri, Arabic – English, vol. 1*. Saudi Arabia: Maktuba Dar us Salam, 1997

115. Kim K-I., Li D., Jiang I., et al. Schizophrenic delusions among Koreans, Korean-Chinese and Chinese: a transcultural study. *Int J Soc Psychiatry* 1993; 39: 190-199

116. Kirov K. A study on the clinic of endogenous melancholy in Bulgarians (in Bulgarian). *Nevrologiya, psihiatriya, i nevrohirurgiya* 1974; 13: 33-38

117. Kirov K. Bulgarian psychiatry: development, ideas, achievements. *Hist Psychiatry* 1993; 4: 565-575

118. Kissinger H. *Diplomacy*. New York: Simon & Shuster, 1994

119. Kleinman A. Do psychiatric disorders differ in different cultures? The methodological questions. In N. R. Goldberger, J. B. Veroff (eds.). *The culture and psychology*. New York: New York University Press, 1995, 631-651

120. Koenig H. G., George L. K., Peterson B. L. Religiosity and remission of depression in medically ill older patients. *Am J Psychiatry* 1996; 155: 536-542

121. Koenig H. G., Huguelet P. (eds.). *Religion and spirituality in psychiatry*. Cambridge: Cambridge University Press, 2009

122. Kraepelin E. *Dementia praecox and paraphrenia* (Kraepelin, 1919, transl. by R. M. Barclay, ed. G. M. Robertson). New York: Robert E Krieger Publishing, 1971

123. Kreiser K. (ed.). *Evliya Çelibi's book of travels: land and people of the Ottoman empire in the seventeeth century; a corpus of partial editions*. Leiden, New York, Köln: Brill, 1996

124. Kring A. M., Gur R. E., Blanchard J. J., Horan W. P., Reise, S. P. The clinical assessment interview for negative symptoms (CAINS): final development and validation. *Am J Psychiatry* 2013; 170: 165-172

125. Kroll J., Sheehan W. Religious beliefs and practices among 52 psychiatric inpatients in Minnesota. *Am J Psychiatry* 1989; 146: 67-72

126. Krueger R. F., Bezdjian S. Enhancing research and treatment of mental disorders with dimensional concepts: toward DSM-V. *World Psychiatry* 2009; 8, 1: 3-6

127. Kulhara P., Avasthi A., Sharma A. Magico-religious beliefs in schizophrenia: a study from India. *Psychopathology* 2000; 33: 62-68

128. Kulhara P., Varma V. K. Phenomenology of schizophrenia and affective disorders in India: a review. *Ind J Soc Psychiatry* 1985; 1: 148-167

129. Lehmann A. C., Myers J. E. *Magic, witchcraft and religion: an anthroplogical study of the supernatural.* Palo Alto: Mayfield, 1985
130. Leonhard K. *Aufteilung der endogenen Psychosen.* 5. Bearbeitete Aufl. Berlin: Akademie Verlag, 1980
131. Lesch O. M., Walter H., Wetschka C., Hesselbrock M. N., Hesselbrock V. M. *Alcohol and tobacco: medical and sociological aspects of use, abuse and addiction.* New York: Springer, 2011
132. Lewis A. "Endogenous" and "exogenous": a useful dichotomy? *Psychol Medicine* 1971; 1: 191–196
133. Lillard A. Ethnopsychologies: cultural variations in theories of mind. *Psychol Bull* 1998; 123: 3–32
134. Littlewood R. DSM-IV and culture: is the classification internationally valid? *Psychiatr Bull* 1992; 16: 257–261
135. Loewenthal K. M. *Mental health and religion.* London: Chapman & Hall, 1995
136. Loranger A., Tulis E. H. Family history of alcoholism in borderline personality disorder. *Arch Gen Psychiatry* 1985; 42: 153–157
137. Marinow A. Prognosis and outcome in schizophrenia. *Int J Psychiatry* 1988; 17, 3: 63–80
138. Matsumoto D., Takeuchi S., Andayani S., Koutnetsouva N., Krupp D. The contribution of individualism-collectivism to cross-national differences in display rules. *Asian J Soc Psychology* 1998; 1: 147–165
139. Mazlish B. *The fourth discontinuity: the co-evolution of humans and machines.* New Haven: Yale University Press, 1993
140. McGlashan T. H. The Chestnut Lodge follow-up study. II. Long-term outcome of schizophrenia and affective disorders. *Arch Gen Psychiatry* 1984; 41: 586–601
141. Messias E., Chen C., Eaton W. Epidemiology of schizophrenia: review of findings and myths. *Psychiatr Clin North Am* 2007; 30, 3: 323–338
142. Mezzich J. E., Kleinman A., Fabrega H., Parron D. L. (eds.). *Culture and psychiatric diagnosis: a DSM-IV perspective.* Washington, DC: American Psychiatric Press, 1996
143. Minkov M. *Cultural differences in a globalizing world.* Bingley: Emerald, 2011
144. Modestin J, Bachmann K. M. Is the diagnosis of hysterical psychosis justified? *Compr Psychiatry* 33; 1992: 17–24
145. Murphy H. B. M. *Comparative psychiatry.* Berlin, Heidelberg, New York: Springer, 1982

146. Murphy J. M. Psychiatric labeling in cross-cultural perspective. *Science* 1976; 191: 1019–1028
147. Murray R. M., Jones P. B., Susser E., van Os J., Cannon M. (eds.). *The epidemiology of schizophrenia*. Cambridge: Cambridge University Press, 2003
148. Namora F. *Deuses et demônios da Medicina*. Lisboa: Livros do Brazil Ltda, 1951
149. Nuller Y. *Paradigms in psychiatry* (in Russian). Kiev: Asocyiacii psihiyatrov Yukrayini, 1993
150. Odutoye K. PTSD: social perspectives and treatment strategies. *Africa Health* 1997; 19: 35–38
151. Okasha A., Maj M. (eds.). *Images in psychiatry: an Arab perspective*. Cairo: WPA, Scientific Book House, 2001
152. Olesen J., Gustavsson A., Svensson M., and the CDBE2010 study group. The economic cost of brain disorders in Europe. *Eur J Neurology* 2012; 19: 155–162
153. Onchev G. Heterogeneity of the possession experiences: a case study from Pemba. *Eur J Psychiatry* 2001; 15, 4: 217–224
154. Onchev G. *Coercion in psychiatry: empirical data and good practice* (in Bulgarian). Sofia: Context, 2010
155. Onchev G., Ganev K. Borderline personality disorder in Bulgaria: period prevalence, syndrome validity, and comorbidity. *Eur J Psychiatry* 2000; 14, 1: 26–31
156. Onchev G., Nikolov I., Kirov G. Paranormal experiences in psychotic patients: results from a descriptive clinical study (in Bulgarian). *Bulletin of the Bulgarian Psychiatric Association* 2005; 13, 1: 4–9
157. Pamuk O. *My name is red* (1998, transl. by E. D. Göknar). New York: Alfred A. Knopf, 2001
158. Paniagua F. A. Culture-bound syndromes, cultural variations and psychopathology. In: I.Cuellar, F. A. Paniagua (eds.). *Handbook of multicultural mental health: assessment and treatment of diverse populations*. San Diego: Academic Press, 2000, 139–169
159. Peralta V., Cuesta M. J. Diagnostic significance of Schneider's first-rank symptoms in schizophrenia: comparative study between schizophrenic and non-schizophrenic psychotic disorders. *Br J Psychiatry* 1999; 174: 243–248
160. Persig R. M. *Zen and the art of motorcycle maintenance*. New York: Bantam Books, 1974
161. Petrov H. *Psychology and psychopathology of the religious feeling* (in Bulgarian). Sofia: Hudozhnik, 1941

162. Pfeifer S. Demonic attributions in nondelusional disorders. *Psychopathology* 1999; 32: 252–259
163. Pichot P. The concept of "bouffée délirante" with special reference the Scandinavian concept of reactive psychosis. *Psychopathology* 1986; 19: 35–43
164. Pöldinger W., Calanchini B., Schwarz W. A functional-dimensional approach to depression: serotonin deficiency as a target syndrome in a comparison of 5-hydroxytryptophan and fluvoxamine. *Psychopathology* 1991; 24: 53–81
165. Popper K. R. *Alles Leben ist Problemlösen*. Munich: Piper, 1994
166. Porter R. *Madness: a brief history*. Oxford: Oxford University Press, 2002
167. Pressman P., Lyons J. S., Larson D. B., Strain J. J. Religious belief, depression, and ambulation status in elderly women with broken hips. *Am J Psychiatry* 1990; 147: 758–760
168. Ramos P. G. Adan JM. Misunderstanding psychopathology as medical semiology: an epistemiological enquiry. *Psychopathology* 2011; 44: 205–215
169. Rashed M. A. Talking past each other: conceptual confusion in "culture" and "psychopathology". *S Afr J Psych* 2013; 19, 1: 12–15
170. Razali S. M., Khan U. A. Hasanah CI. Belief in supernatural causes of mental illness among Malay patients: impact on treatment. *Acta Psychiatr Scand* 1996; 94: 229–233
171. Rees E., O'Donovan M. C., Owen M. J. Genetics of schizophrenia. *Curr Opin Behav Sci* 2015; 2: 8–14
172. Rhi B-Y. Culture, spirituality, and mental health. *Cultural Psychiatry: International Perspectives* 2000; 24: 569–579
173. Riggio R. E., Feldman R. S. (eds.). *Applications of nonverbal communication*. New Jersey: Lawrence Erlbaum Associates, 2005
174. Robins E., Guze S. B. Establishment of diagnostic validity in psychiatric illness: its application to schizophrenia. *Am J Psychiatry* 1970; 126: 983–987
175. Ross C. A. Commentary on positive associations between dichotic listening errors, complex partial epileptic-like signs, and paranormal beliefs. *J Nerv Ment Dis* 1994; 182: 56–58
176. Ross C. A., Miller S. D., Reagor P., Bjornson L., Fraser G. A., Anderson G. Structured interview data on 102 cases of multiple personality disorder from four centers. *Am J Psychiatry* 1990; 147: 596–601
177. Runciman S. *The history of the First Bulgarian Empire*. London: G. Bell & Sons Ltd, 1932

178. Salem D. A., Reischl T. M., Gallacher F., Randall K. W. The role of referent and expert power in mutual help. *Am J Community Psychol*, 2000; 28: 303–324
179. Sartorius N. Quality of life and mental disorders: a global perspective. In H. Katschnig, H. Freeman, N. Sartorius (eds.). *Quality of life in mental disorders*. Chochester: John Wiley & Sons; 1998, 319–328
180. Sartorius N., Gaebel W., Lopes-Ibor J. J., Maj M. (eds.). *Psychiatry in society*. Chichester: John Wiley and Sons, 2002
181. Scaller M., Crandall C. S. (eds.). *The psychological foundations of culture*. New Jersey: Lawrence Erlbaum Associates, 2004
182. Scharfetter C. Schizophrenia ego disorders – argument for body-including therapy. *Schweiz Arch Neurol Psychiatr* 1999; 150: 11–15
183. Schipkowensky N. *Psychotherapy versus iatrogenie: a confrontation for physicians* (Schipkowensky, 1965, transl. from German). Detroit: Wayne State University Press, 1977
184. Schneider K. *Psychopathic personalities* (Schneider, 9th ed., 1950, transl. by M. W. Hamilton). London: Cassel, 1958
185. Schneider K. *Clinical psychopathology* (transl. from German). New York: Grune & Stratton, 1959
186. Sharankov E. *The nestinarstvo: essence and pathos psychophysiological view on fire walking* (in Bulgarian). Sofia: Lekop, 1947
187. Shibutani T. *Social psychology* (in Russian). Moscow: Progress, 1969
188. Simpson M. A. Multiple personality disorder. *Br J Psychiatry* 1989; 155: 565
189. Snezhnevsky A. V. Nosos et pathos schizophreniae. In A. V. Snezhnevsky (ed.) *Scizophrenia. A multidisciplinary study (in Russian)*. Moscow: Medicina, 1972, 5–11
190. Solzjenyicin A. *One day in the life of Ivan Densiovich* (transl. by R. Parker). New York: Dutton, 1963
191. Sperry L., Gudeman J. E., Blackwell B., Faulkner L. R. *Psychiatric case formulations*. Virginia: APA, 1992
192. Spitzer R. L. Psychiatric diagnosis: are clinicians still necessary? *Compr Psychiatry* 1983; 24: 399–411
193. Stanev E. *Antichrist* (in Bulgarian). Sofia: Voenno izdatelstvo, 1970
194. Stankushev T. *Drug addictions* (in Bulgarian). Sofia: Medicina i fizkultura, 1982
195. Stauder K. H. Die toedliche Katatonie. *Arch Psychiatr Nervenkr* 1934; 102: 614–634

196. Steel Z., Marnane C., Iranpour C., et al. The global prevalence of common mental disorders: a systematic review and meta-analysis: 1980–2013. *Int J Epidemiol* 2014; 43: 476–493
197. Stilo S., Murray R. The epidemiology of schizophrenia: replacing dogma with knowledge. *Dialogues Clin Neurosci* 2010; 12: 305–315
198. Stone M. *The borderline syndromes: constitution, personality and adaptation*. New York: McGraw Hill, 1980
199. Stoyanov Z. *Notes on the Bulgarian uprisings. A story of witnesses. 1870–1876. vol. 1–3* (in Bulgarian). Sofia: Bulgarski pisatel, 1977
200. Strauss G. P., Honga L. E., Gold J. M., et al. Factor structure of the Brief Negative Symptom Scale. *Schizophr Res* 2012; 142: 96–98
201. Suhail K. Phenomenology of delusions in Pakistani patients: effect of gender and social class. *Psychopathology* 2003; 36: 195–199
202. Synnott A. Tomb, temple, machine and self: the social construction of the body. *Br J Sociology* 1992; 43: 79–110
203. Szasz T. S. *The manufacture of madness*. London: Routledge & Kegan Paul, 1971
204. Teggin A. F., Elk R., Ben-Arie O. A comparison of CATEGO Class 'S' schizophrenia in three ethnic groups: psychiatric manifestations. *Br J Psychiatry* 1985; 147: 683–687
205. Torrey E. F., Yolken R. H. Psychiatric genocide: Nazi attempts to eradicate schizophrenia. *Schizopr Bull* 2010; 36, 1: 26–32
206. Toynbee A. J. *A study of history* (abridgement of vols I–VI by D. C. Somervell). New York: Oxford University Press, 1947
207. Toynbee A. J. *A study of history* (abridgement of vols VII–X by D. C. Somervell). New York: Oxford University Press, 1957
208. Tseng W-Sh, Streltzer J. (eds.). *Culture and psychotherapy: a guide to clinical practice*. Washington, DC: American Psychiatric Press, 2001
209. Turkle S. *Life on the screen: identity in the age of the Internet*. New York, London, Toronto, Sydney, Tokyo, Singapore: Simon & Schuster, 1995
210. Turner T. H. Schizophrenia as a permanent problem. Some aspects of historical evidence in the recency (new disease) hypothesis. *Hist Psychiatry* 1992; 3: 413–429
211. Tylor E. *Primitive culture: researches into the development of mythology, philosophy, religion, language, art, and custom*. London: John Murray, 1891
212. Üstun T. B., Bertelsen A., Dilling H., et al. (eds.). *ICD-10 Casebook. The many faces of mental disorders: adult case histories according to ICD-10*. Washington, DC: WHO, American Psychiatric Press, 1996

213. Vakarelsky H. *Ethnography of Bulgaria* (in Bulgarian). Sofia: Nauka i izkustvo, 1977
214. Van Praag H. M. Can stress cause depression? *Prog Neuropsychopharmacol Biol Psychiatry* 2004; 28: 891–907
215. Vassilev V. *The medicine in ancient Thrace* (in Bulgarian). Sofia: Medicina i fizkultura, 1975
216. Vlachos I. O., Beratis S., Hartocollis P. Magico-religious beliefs and psychosis. *Psychopathology* 1997; 30: 93–99
217. Waldfogel S. Spirituality in medicine. *Primary care* 1997; 24: 963–976
218. Wessely S., Wardle C. Mass sociogenic illness by proxy: parentally reported epidemic in an elementary school. *Br J Psychiatry* 1990; 157: 421–424
219. Whorf B. L. Science and linguistics. In: J. B. Caroll (ed.) *Language. Thought and reality.* Cambridge: M.I.T., 1956, 247–248
220. Wilson N. G. (ed.). *Herodoti historiae* (1908). Oxford: Oxford University Press, 13th ed., 1976
221. World Health Organization. *Report of the International Pilot Study of Schizophrenia, vol. I.* Geneva: WHO, 1973
222. World Health Organization. *The ICD-10 Classification of Mental and Behavioural Disorders: Diagnostic Criteria for Research (DCR-10).* Geneva: WHO, 1998
223. World Values Study Database. http://www.worldvaluessurvey.org/wvs.jsp (Accessed: 29.11.2017)
224. Yusim A., Anbarasan D., Hall B., Goetz R., Neugebauer R., Ruiz P. Somatic and cognitive domains of depression in an underserved region of Ecuador: some cultural considerations. *World Psychiatry* 2009; 8: 178–180
225. Zhechev T. *The myth of Odysseus* (in Bulgarian, 2nd ed.). Sofia: Prima, 2004
226. Zimmerman M, Ruggero C. J., Chelminski I, Young D. Is bipolar disorder overdiagnosed? *J Clin Psychiatry* 2008; 69: 935–940

Lightning Source UK Ltd.
Milton Keynes UK
UKHW020351280121
377770UK00001B/33